STROKE OF LUCK

MY LIFE IN AMATEUR ATHLETICS

STROKE OF LUCK

MY LIFE IN AMATEUR ATHLETICS

STEVEN KELLY

Heather
With thanks
and best wishes

ROAN IMPRINT

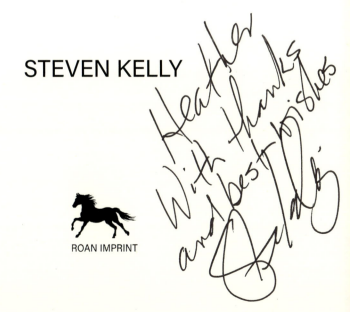

ISBN 978-1-7390380-0-7 (Paperback Edition)
ISBN 978-1-7390380-1-4 (eBook Edition)

Editing by Rona Altrows
Front cover image by Deborah Kelly
Front cover design by Roan Imprint

Published by Roan Imprint
1500 14 St SW Suite 119
Calgary, AB T3C 1C9
Canada

Visit www.mysecondrunninglife.com

To the strong and resilient women
I've been blessed to have in my life:
Mom, Nonna and Grandma, Kathleen and Carolyn,
Lisa, and for always, Deb

Author's Note

This book is a memoir. It presents the author's recollections of certain events and conversations, some of which occurred many years ago. Everything in this book is factual. The author's memory is, however, far from perfect. Some names have been changed to protect the privacy of the individuals involved. Where this has been done, it in no way alters the essence of the story.

Foreword

It was wonderful to read Steve's book. As one of the Foothills Medical Centre Stroke Teams physicians that played a minor role in his care, it is always terrific to learn, several years later, that patients are doing well. The theme of *Stroke of Luck*—the role of athletics and exercise in Steve's life, before and even more so after his recovery—is topical and important.

We all have to move to live. For so many of the ailments that can afflict humans, exercise reduces, sometimes substantially, the chance of those illnesses occurring. When illness does occur, exercise and activity improve recovery or slow the progression of disease.

If Steve's book can inspire others to pursue a more active life, then it will have achieved a key purpose. If it can also inspire builders and planners and engineers to build environments, indoor and outdoor, that promote that physical activity, then whole groups and neighbourhoods will benefit. If it can inspire political leaders to imagine a society where these environments are protected, encouraged, and nourished, then an entire nation can thrive.

The adventures Steve shares in *Stroke of Luck* will be motivational, particularly his accounts of the mountain relays in our beautiful province of Alberta. Demonstrating the importance of a physical lifestyle, members of our medical team participated in the Kananaskis 100 Mile Relay this past June.

My message to Steve and to his readers is the same: Be well and keep running!

— Michael D Hill, OC MD MSc FRCPC FRCS
July 2023

Preface

ON THE SOUTH SIDE of Fiftieth Avenue, between Sixteenth Street and Nineteenth Street, there is a shaded, grassy path that takes the runner past the north end of the Glenmore Athletic Park. Although the park is home to tennis courts, a pool, sports fields of all kinds, and even a velodrome, for me there was only one facility that mattered—the running track. A glance to the south as I ran between the fence and a row of mature poplar trees let me enjoy a close-up view. It made no difference what was going on there as I passed—a track meet in full swing, a few young sprinters working on their starts, or most often, nothing at all. There was something familiar and comfortable about this place. Even when deserted, the perfection of the white lane markings on the red synthetic rubber surface spoke to me of possibilities.

For years, I ran by this spot as a competitor. Just seeing the track invited a quickening of my pace. If I was early into my run, this was the point by which any initial stiffness had been cleared away, and my attention could turn fully to the day's workout. Or if I was heading home and already feeling the exertion of a long run, with tired legs anxious for the finish, I would find myself lifting my knees and leaning forward into my stride. It was as if my muscles had been trained to respond to this visual clue, even without a coach in sight. These were lessons learned long before, and not easily forgotten.

My mind, too, could be taken elsewhere by the sight of the track. Overwhelmed with positive thoughts, I found that memories of my racing heroes often flooded my senses. I might see my brother Paul, cruising powerfully into his final sprint in an 800-metre championship race. Or hear the crowd roar as Steve Prefontaine clung audaciously to his lead in the Munich Olympics 5000-metre final, only to finish out of the medals. I was there too, of course, straining for the finish of my assigned leg in a 4x400 metre relay or doing countless workouts down through the years. Not surprisingly, my feet often seemed to find their own way onto this short stretch of Fiftieth Avenue. After all, many of the happiest moments of my life were spent in places just like this.

I wonder, how can images from half a century ago seem more real than those of the last five years? Yet, it is those latter events—unexpected, frightening and yes, very real—that prompted the writing of this narrative. In a lifetime of experiences, one small event—a single snapshot, as it were—might have easily been overlooked. But in hindsight, I see that some single events possess real power. For a teenager, searching for his place, his experience of one event could change the future arc of his life story. My life story. And so, decades later, with my future not knowable but at least predictable, I should not have been surprised when another episode upended it all.

Now, with full knowledge and greater appreciation of how blessed I am, I need the sanctuary of the grassy path next to the running track more than ever. Fortunately, I can once again lace up my trainers and go for an easy jog between the fence and the row of trees, glance to the south, and invite a flood of positive memories.

Sure, my priorities have shifted. After all, I have traded whatever former interest I had in personal bests and age group race records for less tangible, but equally valid, results. But that is why this story seemed worth telling. While there can be no guarantees in life, there will always be new opportunities for growth as a human being.

My ordeal turns out to have been a stroke of luck.

Calgary Marathon Weekend—May 28, 2017

I WOKE UP BEFORE MY ALARM, with the butterflies already churning in my stomach to remind me that this was a special day. Race day. Even with the hundreds of race days that had gone by before it, this feeling never got old. Race days are different. Vital. Intense. *Authentic.*

That morning, I was entered in a ten-kilometre race—a 10k. It was part of a full weekend of activity, with the Calgary Marathon as the main event. The races would all start and finish at Stampede Park, a short drive from home. The weather was good. It was a beautiful spring day. I checked the forecast for the last time. If it was right, the temperature might be a bit warm for my liking. At least that meant I could be less finicky about my preparations. And besides, for a 10k, I didn't expect to be on the road long enough that the temperature would be a problem. Since Deb was working that day, I would have to get myself to and from the race. Given the conditions, I wouldn't need much support anyway. Her good luck text was waiting for me when I got up.

I had enough time after my usual race-day breakfast to hurry over to the crest of the tough Premier Way hill, a few blocks from my house. There, I watched the lead runners in the marathon as they passed the eleven-kilometre banner. Seeing these incredible athletes in full flight gave me just the boost of motivation I needed. I rushed back home and tossed my small bag in the car. I drove to Mission and parked on a deserted street. As I walked along the Elbow River pathway toward the start area, the buzz of the crowd grew louder. I let the positive energy that always surrounds a race draw me in—the excitement generated by hundreds of runners as they prepared to test their limits in competition. Approaching this scene felt like coming home. Knowing I had put in the necessary work over the winter session, I allowed myself to look forward to a good outing.

I like to arrive about an hour before the start, even though I rarely need that much time to get ready. I would rather take my time and go through my routine, just as I did four decades earlier when preparing for a high school track meet. Inevitably, these scenes of controlled chaos made me think about those days. And that morning, I felt like the teenager I had been as I passed the idle midway and approached the grandstand.

It's not to say nothing had changed. I was feeling quite comfortable with the progress I'd made in preparing for races. It had taken me a long time to get there, but I felt like I now had all the physical and mental tools needed to put a solid performance together. Relaxation is a prerequisite for success, and my well-rehearsed pre-race rituals helped to settle me down.

One thing had not changed. I needed to keep to myself in the final minutes before the start. If Deb had been there with me, I would not have been great company. To be honest, I would have been a pain in the ass. Chalk it up to nerves, the same nerves that were doing their best to undermine my relaxed and ready state. But that morning, on my own, I felt no guilt. I was free to find a quiet spot to sit and get my thoughts together. It was time to visualize the result I expected and to remind myself of one important thing.

"You're ready and you can do this!" I said to myself, under my breath.

I used this time to silently reflect on my race plan. I had agreed with my coach, Janice, on a tactical plan that was meant to give us an early indication of my progress towards my goal for the season—a sub-forty-minute 10k. She was happy that I had committed to a target. It's hard to explain, but I had been somewhat ambivalent about racing for several years. I found that I enjoyed—maybe that was the wrong word—the feeling of achievement that came with structured training. As for racing, I felt I had already accomplished most of my major goals. Still, I was looking forward to the prospect of shorter and more frequent races in 2017. It was a change of focus that had revived my enthusiasm for competition, and this was going to be my first real test.

As Janice and I had decided in our planning meeting, I would see her out on the road at about the 3k mark, and maybe once more at the 7k mark if she could get there in time. The course was flat and fast, an out-and-back circuit just south of the downtown core. It was an ideal course for spectators, and for coaches. I knew the main thing Janice would be watching for was that I didn't overdo it in the first third of the race. This had often been one of my tactical errors.

Whether because of superstition or reality, I felt more prepared if I put my kit on after my warm-up. So, that morning, as on every other race morning, I did an easy, ten-minute jog and then some light stretching, before putting on my club singlet and carefully lacing up my racing shoes. I had pinned my number bib onto my singlet last evening, leaving one less detail to worry about on race morning. I checked my bag. The light feeling of a few brisk strides in my racing shoes reminded me what I was there to do. I adjusted my lacing a little and added a double loop to prevent any mishaps.

I was confident and ready. The butterflies had dispersed. In their place I felt nervous energy coursing through my whole body.

Five minutes before the 9 A.M. start, I purposefully made my way through the crowds and the barricades. I knew exactly where I was heading. I took up a position in the centre of the road, in front of the 2,100 runners who were beginning to assemble on Olympic Way, and right behind the corral set aside for elite runners. Experience told me that this was a sensible decision. With admiration, I watched this small group of fast men and women finish their warm-ups and get themselves into position.

Nine o'clock came—and went.

Eventually, we were informed that the police were working with course marshals to deal with an unspecified issue. We would have to wait for the all-clear. So we waited. And waited. The sun was rising in the sky, and my anxiety about the temperature rose with it. The elite runners did more strides to stay loose, crossing the barrier laid across the road that would hopefully soon be our official start line. I heard the electronic equipment beep as it detected the transmitters affixed to their race bibs. The rest of us had no such option. We were trapped.

I looked around. To my left was a group of mature but inexperienced runners, their brand-new race shirts a sure giveaway. I peeked to see if they had committed the gravest of rookie sins by pinning their bibs on their backs. To my right were several wheelchairs. Not racing wheelchairs, just regular wheelchairs being pushed by aides. How strange, I thought. How dangerous. Behind me were a couple of giggling kids with GoPro cameras strapped to their heads. By chance, I had stood in the only narrow stretch of road where there was little risk of getting caught up in a crash.

For a moment I was struck by how amazing it was to be here, standing at the front of this diverse field. There were runners of all ages and skill levels, and hundreds more women than men. What a change from my early days in the sport. Running really had become mainstream. Sometimes too much so, I decided. I made a mental note to write to the event organizers with some suggestions. But mostly I stewed about the growing delay.

About twenty minutes after nine, we got down to business. I endured the perfunctory speeches from local dignitaries. It felt like I had done my warm-up ages ago. I did some small stretches in place, shaking out my arms and legs to relieve the building tension.

It was only when the gun finally went off that I realized the delay had caused my Garmin to go to sleep. This was a new, high-tech GPS device that I hadn't yet figured out how to use. I tried to get it going while keeping an eye on tripping hazards and the enthusiastic runners around me. Darn! I should have worn my trusty old Timex watch. After about half a block, I convinced the thing to start, and I turned my attention to the task at hand. As we headed west along a normally busy Eleventh Avenue, the sun cast long shadows in front of us, throwing the imperfections on the asphalt surface into sharp relief. I relished the special feeling that always came with displacing cars and drivers from a public roadway.

It was warm. Around me, the field was sorting itself out, as the over-dressed and over-keen began to realize their mistakes. I checked my breathing and my stride, and I tried to ignore what runners around me were doing. I smiled as I thought about the commotion going on behind me.

The first kilometre ticked by almost immediately, and I was reminded of why I liked the idea of running more 10k races. There is plenty of scope for strategic racing, I would have lots of interesting events to choose from, and the recovery times are short. Then I scolded myself for letting my mind wander.

I spotted Janice at the 3k mark, just as we had planned. I was feeling great. I did my best to tidy up my form, hoping to leave her with nothing to criticize. I'm not a runner blessed with ideal technique, although after, who knows, maybe a hundred thousand kilometres, I was as efficient as I was going to get. My pace was on target, a little over four minutes per kilometre. I gave her a thumbs-up.

A left turn on Eighth Street took us south to Seventeenth Avenue. We turned right and headed further west, passing cafes and shops. I stole a glance at diners, who were beginning to look up from their brunch as we went by. I was shocked to realize that these were the first people I'd seen that day who had nothing to do with the race. They didn't even seem to know that it was a race day. Such empty lives!

We reached Fourteenth Street and headed north. I passed the 5k mark in twenty minutes, twelve seconds (20:12)—right on pace. Then, a sweeping right turn onto Ninth Avenue for the return leg, which would take us east past downtown skyscrapers and the Calgary Tower. I gathered myself for the work yet to come, and I moved up another place as the field stretched itself out further.

I had often struggled in the late stages of races, because of a misjudged early pace. Volumes have been written on pacing, and yet little two words—*even pace*—would do. So, with Janice's help, I was determined to execute better. In this, my first race of the season, I had found a good rhythm and was well-positioned, but she wanted me to shake things up with a series of surges—no more than a hundred metres each—as I passed the 7k, 8k and 9k marks.

Janice had walked over a couple of blocks to see me pass on the inbound leg. As I spotted her, she shouted a word of encouragement, and signaled that it was time for my first surge. I responded with a shoulder shrug. What had happened to my confidence? The surges were nothing more than short accelerations, no different than what all those weeks of interval workouts had prepared me to do. The idea was to shake any competitors who might be trying to keep pace with me. I already knew there was no one behind me.

Nevertheless, I followed the plan and drove my arms forward to increase my cadence.

The wave of vertigo came out of nowhere and washed over me as I eased back into my target pace. My head was spinning. The course took a few sharp turns at this point, encircling the curvaceous new building in the East Village that houses the National Music Centre. There were many spectators lining the route at this advantageous location. I heard their shouts swirling around my head. The turns and the noise only added to the balance problems I was already having. I completely lost my focus. I staggered forward. I slowed to an unsteady walk, barely able to set one foot down in front of the other. The vertigo lasted for a block, maybe two, and then it passed. I resumed jogging and cautiously added some pace.

By now, I was heading south on my way back to Stampede Park, for the finish in front of the grandstand. Through the fog that still filled my head, I heard Janice's voice telling me to feel the pull of the finish line. The road dipped briefly down and then back up as we followed the contours of the Fourth Street underpass. How could such a small hill be so painful? The sun was high in the sky and directly in my face now. I was thankful I was wearing a hat. I gave up the idea of any further surges and opted instead for a steady pace to the finish.

I already knew that the last couple of kilometres would be challenging, as we could see the park long before we reached the stadium. It was no longer a struggle to stay upright, but I was certainly straining to make forward progress. My head had cleared enough that I could take a look around for other runners. No one was threatening me. I was holding my own.

I was relieved to reach the final left-hand turn, just north of the grandstand. A quick right-hander revealed the finish line straight ahead. Fighting to hold my form through the fatigue, I crossed the line in a respectable time of 41:15. I was twenty-second overall. It wasn't a perfect result, but it wasn't bad either. Even as I walked through the finish area, picking up some much-needed water, I knew I would have an excellent chance to win my age group. I soon found out that I did win, and by more than four minutes, a surprisingly wide margin. Sometimes things work out.

Janice caught up with me as I sat in the shade and recovered. Tired runners were still trickling across the finish line. Both of us were satisfied with my performance. It was the kind of data point we'd been looking for, something to build on for the season. I had every reason to be confident. There were things I could have done better. I was caught off-guard by the wait on the start line, which messed up my watch. Talk about rookie mistakes.

Then there was the spell of vertigo. I mentioned it to Janice. We agreed it was likely due to the warm conditions, the long delay, and the effect of my brief surge at 7k.

How wrong we were.

Steeltown

I WAS BORN INTO AN unremarkable family, in an ordinary city, in the summer of 1960. I was raised in a working-class neighbourhood by my working-class parents. I was the second of four children in a traditional Catholic family. At first glance, there is little that would have distinguished my family from others in that neighbourhood of that city at that time.

The city, my hometown, is Hamilton, in southern Ontario. To the extent that people think about it at all, they tend to see Hamilton as a rather uninspiring, industrial city. I've come to realize that this is an opinion often formed without much direct experience. Many people have only ever seen Hamilton's least attractive side, its heavily polluted harbour, while passing over the Skyway Bridge on their way to or from Toronto, Buffalo, or some other supposedly more interesting place. But, as a medium-sized city that sits at the far west end of Lake Ontario, Hamilton may be the most Canadian of cities. In much the same way that Canadians often define themselves as not being American, Hamiltonians tend to define themselves as not being Torontonians. Toronto, the big city and the centre of everything, looms over Hamilton about an hour's drive to the east.

Even in Toronto's shadow, Hamilton could still manage some swagger in the early 1960s. For the better part of the next generation, that is to say, my generation, Hamiltonians could take pride in knowing that much of Canada's prosperity was built from the steel produced in the city's prolific mills. Hamilton's nickname, Steeltown, was worn as a badge of immense local pride. But the city's decline had already started. It was slow and unrelenting, like rust on bare steel.

* * *

If you cared to take a closer look, you would find some nuance to my family's story. The Catholic upbringing is challenging enough. Making it often more challenging, and never less interesting, is the straddling of Italian-Catholic traditions on one side and Irish-Catholic traditions on the other.

My mother is Carmela, but this is always shortened to Carm. She once told me she didn't like her name when she was growing up, because no one else she knew had the same name. What a shame. I think her name is beautiful. She eventually came to see it that way too. By any name, Mom deserves first mention and first consideration in my story. She is a saint: strong but flexible, caring but tough when she needs to be, and totally devoted to us. Mom is a second generation Canadian, the daughter of Sicilian immigrants. Her parents, my Nonna and Nonno, Rosa and Giuseppe Celi, were uncomplicated, hard-working people. The story of how they came to be in Hamilton may not be unique, but it is a story of courage and determination, nonetheless.

Giuseppe was born in 1900. In 1923, he left his hometown of Castroreale, a medieval town perched high on a hill in the northeast corner of Sicily. He followed the lead of his older brother by emigrating to Canada. Giuseppe arrived in Hamilton on his own, in search of a better life. Four days later, he found a job at the Steel Company of Canada—Stelco—manually separating iron ore into different grades.

In January 1929, after a suitable match had been arranged with Rosa, a daughter of the Coppolino family, Giuseppe made the long voyage back to Sicily in rough seas. There, he met his fiancée and her family for the first time. They were married on March 31, Easter Sunday, and returned together to Canada in May. Rosa and Giuseppe started their family just as the world sank into depression. They raised four children: my Uncle Tony, my mother and her twin sister Concetta (my Aunt Connie), and my late Aunt Mary. Years later, when my mother and her siblings started families of their own, they all settled within a short distance of the comfortable house on Maple Avenue where they had grown up. That house would become the nexus of family life during our formative years.

* * *

My late father, Ken, was a charming fellow who never seemed to worry too much about anything. In that way at least, he suited the Kelly name—luck of the Irish and all that. And his approach to life may have led you to believe that this was at least partially true. It's hard to know why, as any connection he had to Ireland was so long in the past and so diluted that it would have to be pure coincidence. Maybe it was as simple as having the name Kelly. Still, given his engaging personality, he wore the name well.

Dad was the youngest of five children, with three brothers and a sister. A couple of his brothers, my uncles Charlie and John, achieved some success in life, if success is to be measured by professional achievement. Balancing that out, a couple of his siblings ended up not doing very well. There were rumours about brushes with the law. You might say that Dad was closest to the middle of the road, judging by the trajectory of his life story. He had his share of ups and downs.

Dad's mother, Ann, was born in the United States—Chicago I think, or maybe it was Detroit. Other than that, I don't really know much about her early life. Dad's father's story is better known. Ambrose, known as Brose, was born and raised in rural Southern Ontario. He was one of fourteen siblings. Grandpa's family roots can be traced back to one Hugh Kelly, who left a dreary town in central Ireland in 1826, a place called Monasterevan. I've been to Monasterevan. I could see why Hugh Kelly left there in search of a better life. I find it somehow reassuring that even though he was separated in time from my Italian ancestors by a century, and was leaving from the opposite side of Europe, his reason for emigrating to Canada was identical. Hugh and his young family settled on a wooded parcel in Adjala, at that time little more than a crossroad in Simcoe County. Based on the size of the families that were typical in those days, I could well be related to every Kelly of my generation in Southern Ontario.

* * *

When Mom was in late pregnancy with me, she and Dad were in the process of moving into their house—the same house I grew up in and that she lives in today. Maybe it was the stress of the move, but fate decided that I would arrive early. I was born six weeks prematurely, on a Saturday morning in August. In that summer of 1960, there were already three in my family, Mom and Dad and my sister Kathleen, who wasn't even a year old. I guess I should say four, if I count Dad's beloved German Shepherd, Sam. My brother Paul was born two years later, in June 1962. Then, in August 1965, my late sister Carolyn arrived to round out our family.

The house that Mom and Dad were moving into is in the older

part of Hamilton. It used to be called the east end, although that distinction is less relevant today. Mom still refers to it that way. She would also talk about the north end, as you headed towards the bay. Further east from our house were the towns of Stoney Creek and Grimsby, and if you kept going, Niagara Falls. In between was rich agricultural land that was ideal for growing fruit. Peaches that tasted like peaches. That land is now mainly given over to grapes for wineries. I suppose there is more money in wine than in peaches.

For those who never did get off the Skyway and have a look around, there is a prominent geographical feature, the Niagara Escarpment, that bisects Hamilton east to west. We Hamiltonians always refer to the escarpment as *the mountain*, even though it is, in fact, a shelf. Where the south end of Hamilton should be is instead taken up by the mountain. From their lofty perch, mountain residents could call the whole lower city the north end, and that would not be far from the truth.

The escarpment is about ninety metres high, and the views out across Lake Ontario from the mountain brow are impressive on a clear day. Getting up there from the lower city by car, it is necessary to take one of several mountain accesses, roads that are cut into the limestone face of the escarpment. Even as a kid, I was amazed by those roads. Later, as an engineer, I would appreciate them even more, as they are quite a feat of civil engineering.

Small differences can be exaggerated, like those between the lower and upper parts of Hamilton that go beyond mere geography. By the 1960s, growth in the city's industrial base had already been going on for a century. The lower city had become mainly a working-class area, while upper city neighbourhoods and surrounding cities like Burlington were the suburbs. The term *north end* picked up a negative connotation because of its historic ties to heavy industry.

This distinction would have been real for my parents because their families each had ties to the north end. Mom was born in a modest house on McNab Street, on the fringe of downtown. The house is still there. Her family moved several times and eventually made their home on Maple Avenue, in the house that Nonno was so proud of. Mom's upbringing in an immigrant family brought her face to face with prejudice. There were neighbours who would not utter a word to my family solely because they were Italian. My mother feels blessed to have also made connections with people who became lifelong friends, or whose small acts of kindness were never forgotten, like the neighbour who gave her and her twin sister loaves of freshly baked bread, which was eagerly taken home and eaten with a little olive oil.

Dad's early life is more of a mystery. His family lived on Fairfield Street North, in a rented house precariously close to the steel mills. The house was once pointed out to me, but I couldn't pick it out now. Non-descript is the word that comes to mind, and although it might be a bit harsh, it does seem appropriate for that part of the city.

After my parents married in 1958, they lived for a time in a one-floor apartment in a house not far from downtown. For them to move to a house on Edgemont Street, a street lined with mature trees, must have been quite a step up. Edgemont sits among many seemingly identical streets, each with red, two-storey brick houses on narrow lots. And their new home, with a maple tree in the front and an impossibly large mulberry tree in the back, must have seemed very inviting.

For me, the lower city—Edgemont—was home, and it will be as long as Mom lives there. I could say that Edgemont has changed a lot since 1960. When my parents moved into the neighbourhood, theirs was the youngest family on the block. I can still name all the older people that lived on my street when I was growing up. Even now we refer to those houses, not by their current residents, but by the residents that lived there half a century ago. And now Mom has become the old guard. Things go in cycles, and when you look back over the decades, it makes you realize how time changes everything. At the same time, it changes nothing at all.

* * *

As I was growing up, my world was small. Within a short distance from my house was my entire immediate family, including both sets of grandparents, my school, my church and all my classmates. Having my grandparents so close was a positive influence on my siblings and me. I especially liked visiting Nonna and Nonno. Their house was only five blocks from ours. It seemed that we were always there, whether for family dinners or just to drop in.

Mom would ask me to go over during the summer to cut their lawn, because Nonno had developed angina and was not supposed to exert himself. Instead, he would hover close by, dressed in long trousers and buttoned shirt, his rolled-up sleeves the only concession to Hamilton's oppressive humidity. He pointed out the spots I had missed and brought me drinks and snacks, even though the whole job took less than twenty minutes. Then I would watch his skilled hands, tanned and leathery from a lifetime of manual labour, clean and sharpen the blades of the push mower.

Nonna, who was always in the kitchen, would have lunch ready for me as soon as I was finished. Her hands, too, were strong and highly skilled, but for quite different tasks. She could prepare enough homemade pasta for the whole family, rolling out and cutting ribbons of fettucine on the dining room table. On special occasions, she would prepare uniquely Sicilian treats. At Christmas, she would make *riso nero*—black rice—a regional dessert of Messina, from rice, chocolate, orange and cinnamon. As a kid, I shied away from it. I found its texture strange. But how I would love to have another chance to taste it now.

Big family dinners were organized for many occasions. My

aunts and uncles would be there, and all my cousins. In the early days, the men wore white shirts with thin ties and trousers, and the women wore fashionable dresses, with white cotton aprons to protect them from splattered tomato sauce. We would somehow fit everyone around the dining room table, eating meals that seemed to go on forever. Nonno's patriarchal pride was written on his face.

The sights and sounds of those dinners, the laughing and talking, the tastes and smells, are as real to me today as when I was sitting on Mom's lap. The food was simple and delicious: chicken baked with rosemary, fresh pasta, salads, desserts. Bottles of Nonno's strong homemade wine were plentiful on the table. As kids, we got a drop of wine in a glass, mixed with 7-Up. As we got older, we got more wine and less 7-Up. And because he could, Dad would liberally pour the wine to fill, and refill, his own glass. Everyone took a generous package of leftovers home.

It is the smells that I remember most about that house, smells that changed with the seasons. Tomatoes stewing on the stove and herbs from the garden. My favourite was the smell of fermenting grapes in the fall. Nonno would order grapes by the crate, and they were delivered to the front of the house, in boxes made from thin wooden slats. He and the men would crush the grapes in an ancient press, basically a barrel with vertical wooden staves and a threaded screw affixed to the top. The press would be set up in the centre of the basement floor. Then, the crushed grapes were left for a week or so in open vats to begin the fermentation process. A sweet, glorious smell filled the house.

* * *

At home, the quarters were much closer. To understand how close, it helps to know that my paternal grandparents lived in the house with my parents, my siblings and me. Tight does not begin to describe eight people living in a two-storey house with one bathroom. That explains why some of my earliest memories were of the house being renovated to add two bedrooms in the attic and a second bathroom in the basement.

My grandparents were decent, honest people. They were welcoming if we came upstairs to sit with them and watch television or play a board game. Grandma liked any kind of spectacle and she would often organize outings for us. When we were little, we would be bundled up each November so we could go downtown with her to watch the Santa Claus parade. In the summer, we would make our way to the beach strip, where we would visit the ancient amusement park with its rickety roller coaster. I enjoyed the beach, but I wondered why there were so many dead fish washed up on the sand. Or she would take us to a nearby theatre for a movie. We always rode the city bus to get places. The name of the transit system, the Hamilton Street Railway, made it sound somehow special. I looked for the trains, but all that ever came were buses.

Grandma was a gambler. When my uncles visited, it was only a matter of time until the cards and dice came out. She would struggle to get down onto the floor so that she could organize a craps game in the corner of the living room. Her laugh was contagious. On Grey Cup Sunday, my uncles would organize a pool and make sure we each got a ticket, leaving us to hope that the score would somehow turn in our favour. Even today, so many years later, family gatherings at the Edgemont house seem incomplete without a game of 31 or Ships. I imagine Grandma watching and wishing she could get into the game.

My grandmother lived for these family events, which she would faithfully record with her Kodak Instamatic camera. She snapped candid, off-centre shots of us, crowded into small rooms for all the important occasions. Most of the resulting pictures are long forgotten, but some have permanence because of how well they reveal what our lives were like. One photograph of us in the backyard is my favourite. In it, I am about seven years old and formally dressed, so this must be a picture from my first communion. Six personalities are captured in this one frozen moment.

Grandpa was a curmudgeon, but he was kind with us. He sat in his favourite lawn chair on the veranda, in the shade of a green awning with white stripes, watching the activity on the street through thick, horn-rimmed glasses. He had an endless supply of colourful one-liners, which hinted at his grouchy side and made us laugh. He would watch us play catch. When one of us retrieved the ball after a bad throw, he would yell out in a deadpan voice, "You couldn't hit a barn door if you were sitting on the latch."

The heat and humidity of Ontario summers were unbearable. On the worst nights, sleeping on the third floor of a house without air conditioning was impossible. I would lie awake and wish for a thunderstorm to appear, just to cool things off. During the long, hot days we relied on Grandma's arthritic knee to make weather forecasts. When a storm was imminent, she would round us up to move her house plants down to the front sidewalk, so that they could soak up the rain as it dripped from the edge of the awning.

* * *

My mother's pale hazel eyes are unmistakable in photographs from her youth. Her shy smile hints at her quiet, introverted personality, and tells the story of her growing up during the Depression and the Second World War. She worked as a secretary at Stelco for a while after high school but put aside her own ambitions once she was married. Years later, when we were all grown, she would take a job as a receptionist at a long-term care facility. She soon became indispensable to the staff and residents there. Of course, we knew that would happen because she already was indispensable to us. It was a small step, and one that let her regain some of the self-confidence that had been eroded by too much time and too much worrying about other people.

Mom has handled difficult times with grace and resilience, and she has faced more than her fair share of difficult times. Pain and grief entered our lives when I was in my early teens. This happened in two separate but related ways. At least they are related in my mind. What I know is that nothing was ever quite the same afterwards, and nothing could ever be taken for granted again. Had we crossed some kind of a dividing line, a transition from the innocence of youth to whatever was to come next? I'm not sure. As for my mother, I never heard her complain or shirk from what she had already accepted as her duty. Given her upbringing, I suspect she had never taken anything for granted as it was.

My sister Kathleen and I are close. It has always been that way. She and I are the closest in age, and when we were growing up, she was the sibling I connected with the best. We got along. As kids, we shared a love of reading. Together, we signed up for a summer reading club, and we would often visit our local library, the cozy branch in the house on Kenilworth Avenue. We laughed at the same things. She is thoughtful, introverted, wickedly smart, funny—in a corny kind of way—and kind. Quite simply, she is the nicest person I know.

I was fourteen when Kathleen was diagnosed with an aggressive type of cancer. I came home from school that ordinary day, to find my parents sitting stone-faced in the living room. The diagnosis shattered the veneer of innocent happiness that had existed up to that point.

Kathleen's ensuing fight would last two years. She endured surgery, radiation and seemingly endless rounds of chemotherapy. Week after sickening week, she was injected with the toxic drugs that offered her the chance for life. I was helpless, knowing that I could not change the terms of her sentence. It was the first time that I knew for certain what cruelty was. I felt guilty, for I had been given a free pass to continue enjoying my life. Mom got no such pass. She was by Kathleen's side every minute. It was as if they went through the treatments together. And together, they survived the horrible ordeal.

* * *

In contrast to my mother, the few pictures I've seen of my father as a young man reveal his easygoing manner. That was true later, too. On the surface, he was happy, even gregarious. Below the surface, though, not all was harmonious. Dad did not finish high school, but he was much smarter than his education would suggest. He was the fellow who could be counted on for a ready quip, and was always the first to stand and make a toast or a speech at a family gathering.

And yet, Dad seemed to be searching for something. At home, he was sometimes melancholic and brooding, a trait that I recognize in myself. When he was in a particularly dark mood, he would listen to a scratchy recording or read from his ragged copy of *Cyrano de Bergerac*, a classic tale of a gifted man who experiences self-doubt because of his physical appearance. Cyrano had a grotesquely large nose. While my father's nose was large, it was hardly of Cyrano proportions. Maybe his confidence was more fragile than he ever let on.

It was on this point that Dad's downfall would rest. He would sometimes say about other people, that they were "the author of their own misfortune." I wonder if he suspected that might be his own fate. You see, despite his many redeeming features, Dad was cursed by a common affliction—alcoholism. Like his father and two of his brothers, he was an alcoholic.

Dad's problems with alcohol grew over the years, eventually consuming him and just about killing my mother in the process.

Like a snake, slowly squeezing the life out of its victim, alcoholism was a beast that wrapped itself around my family. In my mind, my father's self-inflicted struggles with alcohol are somehow linked with my sister's illness. It seemed that things got worse after my sister took sick, as if his only way to cope with her suffering was to drink more. Once he was on that path, there was no turning back. And because Mom was the heart of the family, she was the one destined to be the focal point of all the pain and turmoil his behaviour caused. She took this on without a single thought for herself.

I don't remember Dad just for the negative things though. He was a person worth knowing. My earliest memories of Dad—maybe my earliest memories of anything at all—are of us sitting in a sunny spot on the floor playing with the family dog, Sam. My only other memory of Sam is when she was being loaded into the back of a van, never to be seen again. I could tell that my father was heartbroken about that. For years after, he would tell us with a tear in his eye that he had first brought Sam home in the pocket of his overcoat.

My father was inseparable from his newspapers and his stereo. He consumed news voraciously. For years, four newspapers piled up in our house. Early on, he had a console stereo, because that is what audiophiles had in the 1960s. I would sometimes go with him to the tiny hardware store around the corner from our house, where they had a tube tester. I had no idea what a tube did, or why it needed to be tested. I had figured out that if the tubes were glowing, they could make music. It was magic. I loved the smell of sawdust and machine oil and rubber in that store. Later, the stereo died and was relegated to being a piece of furniture. It still sits in a bedroom in the Edgemont house.

In the close quarters of that cramped house, there weren't many secrets. As we four kids grew up, we became more aware of the reality of Dad's addiction to alcohol. For a long time, it was something of a novelty. As kids our first reaction was to laugh at his drinking.

Kathleen and I made jokes about it, maybe because we didn't know what else to do. And besides, Dad, his brothers, and his father would get more animated and louder as they drank more. It was fun when they all got together. For that reason, we looked forward to visits from my Uncle John and Aunt June. They lived close to us and dropped in often. He would hide a box of Smarties for each of us in a pocket or a sock. Alcohol lowered inhibitions, so we would watch as he and Dad become the life of the party.

Reality could be harsh, though. When the next morning came, the crash was complete. All signs of the funny, energetic persona were gone. Hangover morning often coincided with our regular churchgoing. As we walked into the church, made our way to our usual pew, and shuffled in, I remember trying to work things out so that I would not end up next to my father. I did not want to stand and sit and kneel next to him with the stale smell of yesterday's booze wafting from him. I'm ashamed of this memory, vivid and sad, because at any other time I was proud to be my father's son.

* * *

Life did go on, and the nightmare of Kathleen's illness receded into memory. It may be human nature to focus more on times of adversity than on the times when things seem to be going well. To be clear, this *is* a story with a good portion of optimism and happiness. After all, weren't we the embodiment of the promise that had brought my ancestors to this country, the promise of a better life? I'll be forever grateful for that. But there would also be more suffering. My father's chronically destructive behaviour would extract a huge toll. Then, decades later, as if fate had held one cruel twist in reserve, my younger sister Carolyn would be struck down with an eerily similar diagnosis to Kathleen's. In the tough times, I always spare a thought for my mother, knowing that she will gear up for each new struggle in her characteristic way—accepting of the reality of the situation and yet clinging to hope with silent courage. Unfortunately, sometimes the odds are long. Too long, as it would turn out.

Lighting the Flame

WHERE I GREW UP, the steel plants were just far enough away to be out of mind. Sometimes we could detect a slight whiff of sulphur, or hear a heavy, rumbling crash from the direction of the mills. Those noises, which could be felt more than heard, were probably from a raw ingot being dropped somewhere in one of the plants.

Any time we were driven up the mountain, we were reminded of how close home really was to the steel plants. I would look to the north as we climbed the Kenilworth Access, and pick out the steeple of our church, St. John the Baptist, peeking out above the trees. Then, as we got a little higher, the steel mills would come into view. Years later I could recognize the No.1 Melt Shop at Dofasco, after I had spent a summer work term there. At a distance of several miles, the blue-green paint of the mills and their white exhaust plumes had a certain stately beauty.

Our house was little more than a block from the foot of the mountain, so the sheer limestone wall with its lush green cover was a familiar presence. In the summer, the sound of cicadas was almost deafening. We lived close to Gage Park, an urban oasis with historic fountains and majestic trees; and to King's Forest, a large green space in the lower city that was bisected by Red Hill Creek as it ran north off the mountain. Dotted along the escarpment were many spectacular waterfalls. In time, these would become my favourite places to run. After I had moved away, an abandoned CN rail line cut into the side of the mountain was turned into a recreational trail. I think I would have enjoyed running there too.

My area of Hamilton is notable for other things, like the original, the very first, Tim Hortons doughnut shop. My friends and I would occasionally step into the tiny storefront on Ottawa Street for a treat. At that time, Tim Horton was still playing hockey for the Toronto Maple Leafs. That was before his untimely demise at the wheel of his sports car, and long before his name became synonymous with Canada. Whenever I see a long queue inside a Tim Hortons shop anywhere else across the country, my mind goes back to that modest store on Ottawa Street.

* * *

The thought of Tim Horton leads me to the subject of sports, which captured much of my attention when I was growing up. This seems like an odd thing to say, because I wasn't particularly proficient at sports. My earliest sporting memory was of Dad flooding the backyard to make us an ice rink. In good years, the ice was decent enough for us to spend a lot of time outside. Paul and I would play hockey, or all four of us would endlessly circle that tiny patch of ice. We would stay outside until our feet froze, and then scream in pain when they started to thaw. Sometimes we got a bit carried away, sending a stray puck flying through one of the basement windows.

The yard that was large enough for our imaginary National Hockey League games has mysteriously shrunk, when I stand in Mom's kitchen and look out on it now. And the mulberry tree, which got so big that it threatened the neighbours' homes on all sides, has been cut down to a stump. Even so, it is a massive stump that still manages to dominate the yard.

I think of myself as a talented skater, but in reality, I probably wasn't very good. I assume that, as it is with running, the perfection we see in our mind's eye is quite different from what others see.

Later, I got interested in football. That came about from my watching our local Canadian Football League team, the Tiger-Cats, on television. They had a reputation as a fearsome team, and they played a rough, hard-hitting style of football. It suited Hamilton. I fell for their swagger and toughness, and I became a lifelong fan. Today, after decades of disappointing results, all I can say is that being a Tiger-Cats fan teaches a person the importance of being patient.

And there was professional hockey. It was typical for all of us to watch *Hockey Night in Canada* on Saturdays. We crowded into our small living room to watch whatever game was on. Each of us would sit in our favourite spot. Mine was on the floor to the right of the television. The main attraction may have been that Mom often baked a pizza for us while we watched.

I was keen to know all the details of the game. I borrowed a book from the library, called *Hockey, Here's Howe*. It was a thin book by the great Gordie Howe, full of practical information about the game and the rules. Because I knew I would have to return the book, I painstakingly copied excerpts into a school notebook so I would have it as a reference. I was obsessed with the details, even if I couldn't explain why I felt it was so important to know the standard dimensions of a hockey rink or how the referee would signal a holding penalty.

So it was that in May 1970, as an impressionable nine-year-old, I was watching game four of the Stanley Cup finals, between the Boston Bruins and the St. Louis Blues. It was less than a minute into overtime. Bobby Orr rushed the St. Louis net and took a pass from

Derek Sanderson, who was behind the goal line. As Orr directed his shot into the net, to win the game and the Cup for the Bruins, I was in awe. I remember, like it was yesterday, Orr's flying celebration of his goal. I was an instant fan of the Bruins, and I had found my first real sports hero in this young, talented defenseman.

As for my own involvement in sports, I was searching for a place to fit. In my elementary school, many of the boys were active in one team sport or another. I wanted to be like them. I had just started Grade 7 in September 1972, when the Canada-Russia hockey series grabbed the country's attention. Tension built through the month. We knew something important was happening when the entire student body was led into the library, to watch the final game on a small television set that had been set up for the occasion. When Paul Henderson scored the winning goal, we were a screaming, cheering mob. That moment of pure joy, and yes, patriotism, was one of the most exhilarating events of my young life.

Naturally, that winter I decided I wanted to play organized hockey. After all, I had skates and I could skate. All that remained was to assemble the rest of the gear. My best friend John was a talented hockey player. He gave me some of his castoffs—sweat-stained pads that were nearly falling apart. But that didn't matter to me. I bought the few missing bits of gear with my savings. I got myself to the registration session on the bus. In fact, I got to almost all my games and practices that way, because my parents didn't own a car. I regularly hauled my hockey gear onto a bus. I managed to do that for several winters on my own.

Because John was such a good player, he was regularly selected for the local all-star team. More than once, he was the league scoring leader. I would tag along with him and his parents to watch his games. It was entertaining hockey, and John was a thrilling player to watch when he was on his game. If someone hit him or got him mad, he would turn into a beast and score almost at will.

He could be an intimidating presence on the ice. That was fun to watch. It was strange though, because at other times, he was only going through the motions. I would listen to the conversation on the way home, thinking that John must have a switch in his head.

Although I was nothing like the player John was, we would often go to a nearby arena together and play shinny. For a few dollars we could play for hours, until we dragged ourselves off the ice. I would marvel up close at how skilled my friend was, how he owned the ice. I even benefited from his prowess, when he would feed me the puck for a soft goal, boosting my ego in the process.

It must have been my interest in the Tiger-Cats that gave me the idea I wanted to play football. It helped that they won the Grey Cup, at home, in December 1972. Following our tradition, a boisterous gathering of Kelly's watched the game on television. There was much eating, and even more drinking. A prize pool was organized, so there was cheering and despair anytime the score changed. But on that special day, we could hear the roar from Ivor Wynne Stadium as our team scored the winning field goal with no time left on the clock.

We played flag football in elementary school. I made the team because everyone who tried out made the team. I didn't play much. On a cold fall day, I stepped onto the AstroTurf field at Ivor Wynne, the same field my hometown heroes played on, and we played for the city championship. I was sent in when the outcome of the game was beyond doubt. I think we won. Later, I tried out for the high school team, but I was among the earliest cuts. My football career was mercifully short.

I was fascinated by bicycles too. I bought my first bike, a cheap ten-speed, with my savings. The owner of my local bike shop was a soft-spoken Italian immigrant. His name—Domenic Malvestuto—made my mother smile, because, as she informed me, it translated to "badly dressed" in English. From the pictures on the walls of his shop, he had been a formidable racer in his native country. He still carried his athlete's physique comfortably. I would watch as his powerful and confident hands performed minor bike repairs.

Later, my bike was stolen from our garage, and I faced a dilemma. I could replace it with something similar, but by then I had a few more dollars to spend. I wanted a *real* bike, an Italian racing bike. Domenic tolerated my frequent visits to his shop. He patiently explained minute details of the bicycles that were in my price range. In the end, with both of us knowing that he did more for me than he should have, I became the owner—nearly—of a legitimate racing bicycle, an entry-level Bianchi. I say nearly because Domenic let me buy it on instalments. Every month for the next year, I brought in an agreed amount of cash, and he recorded the transaction on the back of my receipt.

Domenic encouraged me to take up riding in a more serious way, even to consider racing. I hesitated, unsure of my own abilities. I found excuses. I convinced myself I would rather just ride with my friends. We did ride together for a while, but it never really caught on. Then Domenic moved to Phoenix, where he became a local hero in that city's cycling community. But through his small acts of kindness, Domenic was already one of my sporting heroes. He personified everything that a sporting hero should be.

I still own the Bianchi. I even gave it a full restoration, after it had sat as a dusty relic in my garage for years. When I was finished the project, and as I was admiring my handiwork, I typed Domenic's name into Google. I learned with shock that he had just died, after a battle with cancer. Had I known subconsciously of his illness, and was that behind my decision to restore the bike, or was it a coincidence? I'll never know. But I will always treasure that Bianchi. I have come to realize that with bikes, I am more taken by the beauty of the machines than by serious riding. Even so, as a nod to Domenic, I could never sell mine.

It was the same when I took turns at golf and tennis, even chess. I wanted to try everything. I even played badminton for a time, although I concede that that one had more to do with its popularity among the girls. Whatever the sport, I think I was looking for was the challenge of trying new things. That, and belonging. I liked the idea of being part of a something bigger than myself, and sports seemed to be the ticket.

* * *

I learned at an early age that if I wanted to participate in any activity, sporting or otherwise, I would have to be self-sufficient. My parents did not have much money to spare. I figured this out from the small stack of twenty-dollar bills that Dad would leave on the dining room table every two weeks, after cashing his paycheque from his job at the post office. Even then, this didn't seem like a lot of money. And it was reduced to nothing when Dad's union would go on strike, as it seemed to do quite often in those days. I realized that Mom must have been very smart to feed us all with this much money, let alone take care of all the other expenses and the extras like the guitar lessons I convinced my parents to let me take. So, I found work and made my own way.

Before I was in my teens, I took a job delivering the local newspaper, the Hamilton Spectator. I toiled six days a week to earn less than twenty dollars. It was worth the effort. I never forgot the invaluable lesson, that having money I had earned brought me a measure of independence. Later, Kathleen got a job at an Esso gas station a few miles from home. She had a friend in high school who worked there. He got her a job and then she got me a job. I think Paul ended up working there too. It wasn't easy working two shifts on a weekend while still in high school, but I stuck with it for a couple of years. I'm not sure which were worse, the strangely quiet night shifts or the hectic day shifts. But I earned sixty dollars a week for my trouble.

* * *

So, as I said, I grew up in a family that would have been indistinguishable from many others of that time and place: families that were dedicated to each other, families that lived by shared values of decency, even some families that dealt with illness and addiction. But it was in my second year of high school that a single event helped determine the course of my life from then on. It happened in gym class, with my interest in sports as keen as ever. The curriculum dictated that we be exposed to a variety of sports. We did something resembling gymnastics, we played lacrosse and soccer, we wrestled. We even tried rugby.

On that September morning, we were being put through our paces by Mr. Menegon, our gym teacher. We were led outside to the football field. There, an unofficial track had been worn into the grass around the perimeter of the field. Our assignment was to run four laps of the field, making a mile, more or less. There was a lot of grumbling from my classmates about this task, which at the time seemed insurmountable.

We all set off, in our white shorts and T-shirts, most of us wearing either tennis shoes or Converse All-Stars. There weren't many true running shoes in those days. After a lap or two, many of the guys were already walking. Not me. I was near the front of the bunch. I remember thinking that this seemed a lot easier for me than for most of my friends. That must have been true, as I was already lapping some of them. I was one of the first few boys to finish.

After we were done, and with kids lying all over the field trying to catch their breath, Mr. Menegon called several of us over. The stragglers were still making their way through the fourth and final lap.

"I want you to meet the cross-country coach here after school," he said.

And just like that, the flame was lit.

* * *

It was ironic that after all my searching for a niche, running found me instead. Maybe the why and the how of the process that brought us together do not really matter. Maybe I should just be content that it happened at all and leave it at that, because many things—everything—seemed to make more sense after that point. It was as if the threads of my personality were suddenly woven together and given a purpose. It was as if I had been handed a tool to help me deal with the burdens my family was only beginning to grapple with.

As I walked over to the starting line on that field on that morning, I had for the most part become the person I was destined to be. And yet, I was about to be changed by the events of the next few minutes—changed in profound and lasting ways. In thinking about how and why that happened, I naturally think about my parents, and how much credit they deserve for putting me on the right path to begin with. There are certain traits that make me who I am, and it is a relatively straightforward matter to connect those same traits in my parents and their parents to my own personality. Even so, I can't help but wonder, how much different a person would I be today if I had not stepped onto that field and run a mile? I believe that there was some synergy between my character and an ingredient that had, until that moment, been missing.

I did bring a few things with me onto the field that morning. Curiosity was the trait that had led me to try all those sports and activities. I believe my curiosity originates from the distinct influences on the Italian and Irish sides of my family. Dad was a curious person, and no doubt that had an influence on me. For his time and place, he had diverse interests, and he was open and accepting of people who were different. We thought nothing of it. While my father never had the same opportunities to travel that I've had, he was passionate about knowledge, whether that came from listening to foreign radio programs or reading obscure books. He never discouraged people from being themselves, and in his circle of friends were some characters who did just that.

I didn't know it at the time but running would add a new avenue of exploration to satisfy my own curious nature. There is no end to the learning that comes from this sport, which challenges the body, the mind, and the spirit. It was to become the ideal diversion for me, and my constant refuge.

I also brought tenacity to my newest pursuit. Even as a child, I gravitated to task-oriented work, and I liked to understand small details. That is probably why I eventually chose engineering as a career. Without a doubt, this dedication came from Mom's influence. I need look no further than the sacrifices her parents made, arriving in Canada as poor immigrants. Or at the hardships she overcame for our family. Her devotion showed up in a thousand unspoken ways, and it still does, but it amounts to the same thing—the resolve to complete the task she had taken on, to raise her children and grandchildren. She did so while taking on more than her share of the responsibility and dealing with more than her fair share of adversity.

Mom's influence has shaped my own worldview. The best I can ever hope for is to follow her example and to put into practice the lessons she taught me. In my own life, I have applied myself to work and leisure pursuits with a dedication that can border on obsession. I've learned that this is not a common trait; not everyone can manage it. Being able to narrow my focus and see a task to completion has gotten me through many tight spots. And once I got involved in running, I would find a practical outlet for my dedication. The process of training and competing for a goal race could be seen as nothing more than a series of small tasks, laid out in front of me, a prelude to reaching the finish line of the race itself. It helps to have a personality that can cope with that kind of structure and granularity.

Perhaps most important, was humility. My parents both had modest upbringings. I know that shaped how they viewed the world, and how they raised us. Mom, especially, never seeks the spotlight. Rather, she avoids it. Dad was different. His personality was more prominent, more visible, because he enjoyed a laugh and could be counted on to make a joke that captured the feeling when we were all together. Still, he often poked fun at himself.

The lesson I try to remember as I go through life is the importance of modesty. I know that I am not the world's best father, engineer, runner, or anything else. But by emulating my grandparents and my parents, who sought nothing more than a better life for their family, I can try to be incrementally better today than I was yesterday. For me, this means being ready to say three little words: "I was wrong." There is always more to learn and we should always strive to improve. I would come to learn that running has a way of providing immediate and sometimes brutal feedback, which neatly reinforces that lesson.

So that's it, to the extent I have any formula for living: be curious, be diligent, be humble. And, of course, run.

More Warning Signs

IN JUNE 2017, I began to experience some strange physical problems. First, there was a peculiar and recurrent problem with my vision. Imagine a glass prism, about the width and length of your index finger. Now, as you are sitting, perhaps as you look at your computer screen, imagine that this prism is parked in your field of vision, at about the ten o'clock position. Then, imagine that the prism is very slowly rotating.

When this first happened to me, I assumed that the fluorescent bulb over my desk was acting up. Switching it off and on did nothing to stop the prism from appearing again. I rubbed my eyes and cleaned my reading glasses, but to no avail.

The mysterious prism made an appearance several times over the course of a few weeks. Each time, it sat there, turning slowly, for about ten or fifteen minutes. Then, just as strangely as it appeared, it went away.

Other odd things happened too. One day in early June, as I was sitting in my office, I had a sensation of fainting in my chair. I felt myself getting heavy, in an out-of-body sort of way, as if my body no longer belonged to me. I was aware of what was happening, but I could do nothing about it. For several minutes I was unable to move. I thought about trying to call out to someone for help, but I was not even sure I could do that. It was as if my brain had disconnected itself from my body. Maybe someone will come and find me, I thought. Then, just like the prism, the feeling subsided and I was back to normal.

I treated these as isolated incidents. My first reaction was that they were somehow the result of pushing myself too hard in an interval training session or a long run. For that reason, I did not mention the problems I was having to anyone. I certainly did not call my doctor to schedule an appointment. What would she have concluded from these strange symptoms? After all, I figured it would be months before I got to see a specialist, if I could have convinced her to make an appointment for me.

While this was going on, I continued to train as I normally did. Deb and I spent a few happy days in New York City, in mid-June, to celebrate her sixtieth birthday. We had been to New York several times, and we preferred to stay in midtown Manhattan, the heart of the city. We enjoyed being close to the museums and the galleries, and of course, Central Park. For this trip, we stayed at the Carnegie Hotel, across the street from Carnegie Hall and three blocks south of the park. We made sure to incorporate a morning run into our daily schedule.

Because our training paces were different, we walked over to the park and back to our hotel together, but we each ran on our own. My spring training program was geared to getting me ready for the 10k races I had committed to. I was scheduled for a tempo run (a run with a sustained section at a fast pace) and a strenuous interval session during our brief stay in the city. For those workouts I could use the long, paved pedestrian path to full effect, reaching the north end of the park before returning to Columbus Circle where I would meet up with Deb.

I did my interval workout on a warm, humid morning, using the countdown timer on my watch. The intervals and rest periods were multiples of ninety seconds. This was a workout where time was more important than distance, so all I needed to do was listen for the beeps—one for a minute thirty, two for three minutes, four for six minutes—to get me through the session. The repetitions lulled me into quiet contemplation of my own thoughts as I ran through the tranquil park. It was a pure expression of the perfection of running: fast, jog, fast, jog, fast, jog. I finished my sets feeling quick and efficient. It was another incremental step on the path of preparing myself to handle the stresses of the upcoming season. I did not even think to carry identification with me while running. I only realized later what a bad idea it was not to.

* * *

During this time, my friend Mahedi and I continued to build on our recent reunion. We had first met fifteen years earlier, when we trained together at Lindsay Park, a large community sports facility with a 200-metre indoor track. Initially, we were led through weekly interval sessions by Ray Croteau and Gord Hobbins, two well-known figures in the Calgary running community. After Ray and Gord stepped away from the sessions, Mahedi took over as coach. By then, we had become close friends and we often trained together.

I have been lucky throughout my running life to find several training partners whose personality and talent were a close match for mine. Mahedi is one of those people. We just click. Whenever we got together to run, it felt right. Much of our connection was unspoken, as our running was our bond. But more important than that, he is a warm and caring person.

After a long hiatus, Mahedi and I were back running together in the spring of 2017. He had reached out to me after overcoming a nagging knee injury and suggested we get together again. Naturally, I agreed. Our regular meeting spot was Edworthy Park in the city's northwest, where we could do hill training, a long run, or an interval workout, as our training schedules dictated.

Through May and June, we ran together often. It never occurred to me to mention the strange prism in my field of vision, or my other symptoms. Besides, if I had any concerns about something not being right, I felt like these had been dispelled by my performance in the annual Kananaskis 100 Mile Relay, known to Alberta runners as the K–100. The race is a one-day, ten-stage relay in Kananaskis Country, a large provincial recreational area just west of Calgary.

Some runners sign up for the K–100 every year. Not me. I enjoyed the race, but I tended to be a bit more cautious about committing to a team. No question about it, I'd had some reasonable success in this event, both with club teams and with corporate teams when I'd worked for Shell Canada. What I like most about the K–100 and other similar relays is the teamwork and camaraderie. It makes me think of what it must be like to organize a mountain-climbing expedition in the Himalaya. Getting a large team of runners organized, with logistics, timing and all the contingencies for weather and traffic, is a monumental task.

I had good reasons for my cautious approach. I tended not to commit to a relay team until close to race day. I could usually be convinced to run if a competitive team needed a spare—there were always spots available—and if I were feeling confident in my ability to run well. That seemed to be a safer position than committing to a team, months beforehand, only to suffer an injury and not be able to run. It had become a fact of life that even though injuries were thankfully still rare for me, they were becoming more common.

Initially, I declined a couple of invitations to run in the 2017 relay. As I might have predicted, my club, Adrenaline Rush, found itself with two teams entered and with runners dropping off for various reasons. The first request to run as a spare came to me, and I deftly (but somewhat reluctantly) deflected it to Mahedi. I knew his conditioning was good, and that he was usually keen to help a local team, but since he had been observing Ramadan for the past few weeks, he wasn't eating any food during the day. To ask him to compete while he was fasting felt to me like I was complicit in a plan to cause him personal harm. I put Janice in touch with him, figuring he was old enough to speak for himself. I soon heard back that he had decided to run with our team.

Mahedi proposed to Janice that he would run Stage 5. It is widely feared as the toughest of the ten stages in the relay. Stage 5 takes runners to the highest point of the Highwood Pass, gaining 450 metres over eighteen kilometres. Mahedi is something of a specialist on this stage, having run it many times over the years. In 2017, Ramadan would end on race day. How he could even consider running such a challenging stage on no food was a mystery to me.

Then another, more urgent, request came in.

"Now we need you too!" read the text from Janice.

I bowed to the pressure and said yes, knowing that I had no real excuses. I had run that decent 10k in late May. Again, I did not mention the vertigo or the other issues I was having. And why would I? I asked Janice to put me on Stage 8, because I knew this stage well and I liked it. It is reasonably demanding, with some rolling hills but a slight net downhill over its sixteen-kilometre length. I figured I had some leverage, as she needed me to run. She agreed.

Deb was to be off work on the day of the relay, June 24, so we made plans for the three of us to go to Kananaskis together, she and Mahedi and me. We would support each other and Deb would drive. It would be a long day, but a worthwhile adventure.

As I was warming up before the start of my stage, I snapped at Deb's efforts to engage in light conversation. I think Mahedi understood that I was feeling the stress and he left me alone with my thoughts. I marvelled at how relaxed and fresh he looked, having completed his gruelling stage just an hour earlier.

My worry about how I would do turned out to be unwarranted. I felt good from start to finish, running a steady pace and a smart stage. Because I had run Stage 8 in 2012, I had instant feedback about how my 2017 result stacked up against my previous performance. I was happy to have run faster than I had five years earlier. It was another positive omen for the season ahead. Both Adrenaline Rush teams in the relay did very well. My team finished first in the Masters' 50 and over category. It was always fun to spend the day with my talented teammates, even if my nerves did sometimes get the best of me.

A few days later, Mahedi and I started a two-set hill workout at a location popular with local runners—the long hill on Twenty-ninth Street, next to the Foothills Medical Centre in the city's northwest. Neither of us felt up for such a workout, so I was agreeable when he asked to cut it short after one set. Fatigue from the weekend was still a factor, so we called it a day and thought nothing more of our decision.

* * *

July 1, 2017—Canada Day—should have been a big deal, as it marked the 150th anniversary of Canadian confederation. Instead, the celebrations were quite lame. The main event in Ottawa was hampered by rain, massive delays due to security checks, and a lacklustre feeling about the whole affair. I watched a bit of the coverage on television, but I soon got bored and switched it off.

The significance of the anniversary made me think about my father spontaneously banging pots and pans at midnight on Canada's centennial, on July 1, 1967. I wondered whether anyone had done the same thing this time around. Probably not, I decided. It had been a different and more innocent time when Canada celebrated its 100th anniversary. I pondered the many changes in society since then, not all of them positive. Then I realized, with a tinge of sadness, that I could clearly remember things that had happened fifty years earlier.

At least I could still run. Since Deb was working all weekend, I had the time to myself. The highlight of my schedule was a long run with Mahedi on Sunday, July 2. I was concerned about the forecast, which called for temperatures of 30 degrees Celsius. What was worse, we started our run late in the day, and the temperature was already high and climbing. As we ran east from Edworthy along the north side of the Bow River, we found ourselves surrounded by families, dogs, and cyclists, all out for the holiday weekend and all attracted by the sun and the warm weather.

The temperatures that were so appealing for everyone else were not so good for us runners. Well, me at least. Mahedi and I have endlessly debated this point. He was born and raised in Tanzania, and because of his east African constitution he prefers warm weather. In fact, anything below 10 degrees Celsius is a problem for him. For me, a lifetime of running in Canadian winters had programmed me for cooler weather. My least favourite conditions for running are (in order): heat, wind, and heavy rain. So, on that day, I would be dealing with my enemy number one.

As we continued to weave in and out along the pedestrian path, dodging strollers, animals, and stray kids, I found myself getting disoriented and dizzy. I was carrying water, but I was already parched. As we approached Calgary's iconic new Peace Bridge and our planned stop at the downtown Eau Claire Y, about seven kilometres from the start, I had another bout of vertigo, just like the one I had during the race in May. I stumbled across the bridge. Mahedi was waiting for me on the south side.

"Mahedi, I have to stop. I just had a spell of vertigo," I said.

Mahedi understood. “No problem, Stevie. Let’s do an easy jog to the Y,” he suggested.

Given the conditions, we decided that I had not taken in enough water. The feeling of vertigo had passed by the time we reached the Y building. Even so, I made sure to drink lots.

When we got back outside, I was already feeling better. We even continued farther east to the next bridge, before crossing back over to the north side of the river for the long return to Edworthy. Several times, Mahedi proposed that we slow down, or even walk. I knew he would walk all the way back with me, should that have been necessary. That is the type of friend he is. But I had no interest in that idea—I had other plans for the rest of the day—and we resumed running, eventually getting back to something close to our ordinary training pace. I didn’t feel great, but I was getting it done.

The cumulative effort of the run eventually got the better of me. At Crowchild Trail, about eighteen kilometres into our run, we caught up with Mahedi’s wife Zuby. She had joined us at the start, as she was in the habit of doing. She would walk the same route that we ran, turning around based on our guess of the time when we would return. If we planned things well, we would all arrive back at Edworthy about the same time.

On this day, we exchanged a few pleasantries with Zuby before carrying on—Mahedi, running as smoothly as ever, and me hobbling behind. I was done, and I knew it. I was reduced to a walk, maybe better described as a shuffle, for the last kilometre or so back to the car.

I would later hear from Mahedi that when we passed her, Zuby had noticed something that she mentioned privately to him.

“Something is wrong with Steve,” she told him.

Zuby is a perceptive woman.

Stoking the Flame

NOW THAT RUNNING HAD CHOSEN ME, it was my turn to learn what it was all about. At fifteen, I was an open book. The cross-country coach I dutifully reported to on that fall afternoon was not a teacher at my school—I'm not even sure what his connection to the school was—but he became a constant presence there. Mr. James had a stern disposition, and a personality that demanded our respect. He met us every afternoon after school and often on the weekends. He was dedicated to the task of turning us into runners, and he knew what he was doing.

We benefited from a program that was well ahead of its time. Mr. James had been a good sprinter and looked like he could still run a formidable 400-metre race. He had learned valuable lessons about athletics training, and as a gifted coach he was able to convey those lessons to us. We did interval training one or two nights a week, tempo runs and long runs. When the weather was bad, we would run circuits of the stairs and hallways inside the school. Even forty years later, when my running schedule called for twelve repeats of 400 metres, I would instantly be transported back to high school for one of our core workouts.

Mr. James saw to it that we gained valuable competitive experience. We ran cross-country races in the fall, indoor track in the winter and outdoor track in the spring. Road races were springing up everywhere and we ran those too. It was not just about running races, but also how to prepare and recover from them. At track meets, we were each signed up for different races because our coach wanted us to experience all of it. We learned how to pass a baton, and we practiced often, so we could run the relay events. We got used to running several track events in a day.

We did more than just run. We lifted light weights. Sessions of basketball or soccer kept us from getting bored. Today that would be called cross-training, but for us it was a fun way to hang out together. I was getting what I craved most, a team sport that I wasn't terrible at. My teammates and I become great friends, as we trained together and travelled to competitions.

Coincidentally, the world around us was discovering running at the same time we were. The mid- to late-1970s marked the beginning of what is now called the running boom. Frank Shorter's win in the 1972 Olympic Marathon for the United States is often cited as the beginning of the boom, but I wonder how strongly that event resonated in Canada. If we were following any world class distance runners, it was more likely to be the top Canadian, Jerome Drayton, or even some of the top British runners like Ron Hill, rather than the celebrated American.

From my perspective, as a kid who was getting caught up in the sport, high school athletics were still the domain of skinny kids like me. Road races, particularly any serious events that were longer than a few miles, mainly appealed to gaunt, sinewy veterans. Things were starting to change, though. Running was becoming more accessible and more accepted. Even if it had not yet reached the status of a mainstream sport, it was becoming more commercial. Guys started showing up at races to sell curious-looking shoes out of the trunk of their car. The shoes were called Nike Waffle Trainers, and they were unlike anything we had seen before. For most of us, they were an expensive novelty. One of my teammates worked in a running shoe store in Hamilton, one of the first independent stores of its kind, and he could be counted on to bring the latest shoes to practice. The rest of us made do with whatever athletic shoes we had. But even that was changing, and we soon started seeing purpose-made running shoes from companies like New Balance and Adidas.

I gave up pretending with other sports because I was willing to go all-in with running. I wondered how I had missed this idea, as I had tried and failed at other sports. Even though I had persevered with organized hockey for a few years and enjoyed it, by the time I turned sixteen it was clear that the differences in skill between me and the best players were just too great to overcome. No one cried over my decision to quit.

Besides, I was beginning to experience the liberating power that running can have. I came to realize that when I was running on my own through King's Forest or Gage Park, there was no need for anything else, or for anyone else. The attraction of running goes well beyond the mere physical action, the mechanical process of locomotion, but it does start there. An efficient runner can be beautiful to watch. For most of us, and certainly for me, that was an ideal that could not be achieved. We can only work with the physical gifts we have been given, so the observant eye of a good coach was invaluable. Mr. James helped us correct the worst flaws in our running posture, and he opened our eyes to the other benefits that running could bring.

My connection with running was revealing itself to be quite complex and nuanced, so a more accurate term for this process may be *discovery* rather than *learning*. The physical side of the sport was what we focused on first, but the important connection for me, and the one that was to deepen over time, was emotional. There was a passion, an internal flame, which came from being involved with the sport. It started with a feeling that when I ran, I was in control. It truly did feel that I had managed to light a flame that came from somewhere within me. I didn't know yet how bright the flame could be, but I had started to explore my potential.

There was more. I began to observe, as I still do, that runners tend to be interesting people. And beyond my shared interest with other runners, there was the rich history of the sport, and the personalities of the great runners. It all combined to make running a unique and special activity. Of course, in the early days, I was only scratching the surface. All I knew was that I wanted more. My growing commitment was the natural result of applying those three personality traits that I brought with me to the sport—curiosity, diligence, and humility.

I found myself being swept up into this new world of athletics. I had paid only passing attention to the 1972 Olympic Games and Shorter's marathon victory. At that time, I still preferred hockey and football. And I mainly remember the Munich games for the wrong reason. Dad watched the NBC television news every evening. Instead of great sporting achievements, we watched in disbelief as hooded terrorists took the Israeli athletes hostage.

By 1976, my perspective had changed completely, in line with my newfound passion. I couldn't wait for the start of the Montreal Olympics. Because the games were in Canada, there were efforts to stoke public interest and to raise money to pay for them. I only cared about the athletics events, and I needed no encouragement. I idolized the middle-distance runners, who combined unbelievable speed with power, and the long-distance runners, who had bottomless reserves of endurance. I waited impatiently for the marathon, by tradition the last event of the games, and I watched as an unknown East German runner, Waldemar Cierpinski, beat the favourite, Shorter.

I learned about the world's other major marathons—Boston, New York, Fukuoka—and about the top long-distance runners. I watched the scarce television coverage of athletics, mostly through the US-centric lens of *Wide World of Sports* on Saturday afternoons. I was captivated by the graceful and likeable Bill Rodgers, the American record holder, who seemed to be floating as he cruised along at sub-five-minute miles. And there was Drayton, an enigma behind his dark shades. He seemed tough as nails, and not as easy to warm up to. I marvelled at reports of their unbelievable training mileage. They both took their places as my sporting heroes, along with other emerging track stars, next to Orr and Malvestuto.

* * *

It seems odd to say it, but despite my youthful enthusiasm for running and racing, it was not a sport that I excelled at. If I am totally honest with myself, I can admit that I was not even very good at it. Whatever success I was to have later was due to a willingness to commit myself to the necessary hard work.

At the time, I think Mr. James was hopeful that he had found a runner with potential. As I walked to the start line of my first 800-metre outdoor race, I nervously asked him how I should run the race.

"Run the first lap as fast as you can and speed up for the second," he told me.

That was simple enough. I tried to do as I was told, because I had bought into his system, and I didn't want to disappoint him. The result was nothing exceptional. I ran 2:07 and finished in the middle of the field.

There was to be a track star named Kelly. It just wasn't me. Mr.

James would have to wait a little longer for him to arrive on the scene. As for me, I'm not sure I ever bettered that first 800-metre time. I could not explain why, and it didn't even matter. The lessons to be learned were still available, and as a keen student, I tried to absorb as much as I could.

We took on challenges that changed with the running seasons. Cross-country season called for trail work on our home course at King's Forest. We got to know every inch of the trails. The long, uphill, fifteenth hole of the golf course that was adjacent to the park where we met after school was a frequent location for our hill training sessions. Sometimes, for variety, our coach would find another steep path up the side of the escarpment to test our fitness.

The indoor track season was a chance to apply our base of fitness to shorter distances. Meets in those days were often held on temporary wooden tracks, set up in venues like the Armoury in downtown Hamilton or Maple Leaf Gardens in Toronto. For us, this was a new and unforgettable experience. It was exhilarating to feel the spring of the boards as we sprinted around the banked corners.

The outdoor season was the pinnacle of the athletic calendar. We prepared for meets and hoped for enough success in the city finals that we could move on to the Ontario championships. For me that wasn't usually in the cards. I simply did not have the raw speed necessary to compete at the shorter track distances. I was content to run at the city meets and support my teammates. After my flirtation with the 800-metre distance, Mr. James was still looking for my specialty. That meant that I was given the opportunity to run some events that others may have avoided, like the steeplechase. I ran a lot of 4x400 metre relays. I ran 3000 metres. Whatever the race, it was thrilling to be there, to be part of a team and to continue exploring my own potential.

Then there were the road races. We drove all over Southern Ontario to run in local events—Toronto, St. Catharines, Guelph.

There seemed to be a race every weekend. We were given ample opportunity to try different distances and race tactics. A faded picture from the Hamilton Spectator shows a wall of us at the start of the Cathedral High School Junior Boys' race. We took up the entire width of Main Street and were dwarfed by the downtown buildings that towered behind us.

I only need to look at the bibs I saved from those races to know that it was a different era. Some races were run to honour historical greats, but I'm sure none of us knew or cared who Lucky Stewart was. The distances were sometimes odd, like 3½ or 1¾ miles. And the bibs were even stranger—hand-scrawled numbers on the back of surplus vinyl wallpaper or bits of cardboard. Finishers' medals? Forget it. We were satisfied if we got a can of pop and a slice of pizza.

Thinking about road race distances reminds me that when I started in the sport, metres were for tracks and miles were for roads. The US was a holdout, gamely sticking to mile distances, even on the track. That meant 2-, 3- and 6-mile races were still common there, even in the late 1970s. I was one of a small cohort of kids who had learned both imperial and metric systems in elementary school, because Canada was transitioning from the former to the latter, and it was thought that we should know how to convert between the two. In retrospect, that might be the single most useful thing I ever learned in school. I have watched road races migrate from 5- and 10-milers to almost all metric distances. Except, of course, the marathon. That has stubbornly stayed at 42.195 kilometres since being set in 1921 by the International Amateur Athletic Foundation. If you prefer imperial units, that is 26 miles and 385 yards, or 26.2 miles. To this day, I still check my intermediate times during races—my splits—in minutes per mile.

* * *

I made progress as a runner through my third and fourth years of high school. I ran through the summers to make sure I would arrive ready for the fall cross-country season. I was learning perhaps the most valuable lesson of all, that there are no secret paths or shortcuts to success in distance running. The program Mr. James put us through started with kids having a degree of talent, but it depended most on a commitment to do the work—the constant work—required to turn us into athletes. I brought the minimal amount of talent, to be sure. What I was willing to contribute was dedication to the program and a degree of tenacity that I didn't even realize that I had at the time.

A solo sport that offered all the benefits of a team sport suited my personality. I felt myself growing in confidence, as I formed the bonds of friendship and common purpose with my teammates. We gave everything in our workouts, day after day, and learned about each other's strengths and weaknesses. We believed in each other. We had fun together, and in the process, we forged ourselves into a team.

That is not to say that commitment alone could overcome differences in individual talent. When my brother Paul arrived at high school, I learned that the talent distribution in my family was far from uniform. He had an intensely competitive personality, as well as natural athletic ability that he was able to seamlessly transfer from one sport to another. The high school football and basketball coaches had been salivating over his arrival for months, since he had single-handedly carried his elementary school teams to multiple championships in those sports.

With my encouragement, Paul came to a cross-country tryout. As a one-year veteran, maybe I thought I could show him the ropes. He did give running a try and he never looked back. He began winning races immediately. How disappointed those other coaches must have been when he took a sharp turn into athletics.

At that time, the idea that a gifted athlete would choose athletics over football was probably heretical. Paul was to become the core, the key ingredient, in a minor dynasty that Mr. James would build for our high school athletics program.

* * *

That same year, Mr. James proposed that several of us tackle a unique challenge, the annual Around the Bay Race in Hamilton. Even now it would seem odd to put young teenagers through the kind of training needed to attempt this road race. Our coach's logic was sound—he wanted us to build a base of fitness for the longer track races.

The Bay Race is billed as the oldest race in North America, and despite a few ups and downs in its fortunes it is a fixture in the city. In the late 1970s, the race was something of a local curiosity. Then, it was named in honour of Billy Sherring, a Hamilton native and one of Canada's great marathoners at the turn of the century. The race distance had changed over the years. In 1977, it was 19 miles and 168 yards, which made no sense in either imperial or metric units. By either measure, it was a long way.

Three of us were signed up for the race, which was held every year in late March. Our training program was simple but surprisingly effective. A couple of times each week, Mr. James would drive us eight or ten miles from the school and drop us off, and we would run back.

Weather is always a potential factor for the Bay Race. On the morning of March 26, it was cool, with a light breeze from the north. It could have been much worse. I was upset to learn on race morning that Paul had borrowed my one and only long-sleeved shirt, the one that I had planned to run in. I was forced to go with a short-sleeved T-shirt under my singlet, and shorts. I wore my newest, prized possession—a pair of orange Tiger Jayhawk racing shoes.

The starting field on John Street in downtown Hamilton consisted of several hundred sinewy veterans of the race circuit, and us. These were the *hard men* of the sport. As a sixteen-year-old, I had no idea what I was about to experience. I had never run a race remotely as long as this one. I was nervous as hell and the butterflies were busy in my stomach that morning. Anticipating our anxiety, Mr. James had driven us around the course a few days earlier.

We set off under grey skies, appropriate for a race that skirts the industrial heart of Hamilton. The first third of the course, heading east along shabby Barton Street, set a dreary tone. We continued east on Burlington Street, with the steel plants and other heavy industries looming over us on our left.

We made our way to Beach Boulevard, for a long flat stretch that offered only a slight improvement in scenery. This natural barrier between Hamilton Harbour and Lake Ontario was desolate and rundown. While I had retained fond memories of summer days on the same strip of beach with my grandmother, it presented a much different picture when running there in late March. The moderate winds, of no consequence at the start, were a much greater test when running along the exposed beachfront. Step for step beside me was my teammate. Andrew was a talented runner who had started into athletics at the same time as my brother. Our other teammate had dropped out somewhere in this section. Andrew and I suffered together, each of us in our own world. Occasional glimpses of whitecaps on the steel blue water of the lake were unnecessary reminders of the harsh conditions. We ran on.

The last third of the race passes through an upscale residential area of Burlington. We knew that this part of the course would bring another set of challenges. Rolling hills on North Shore Boulevard were notorious for wearing down already tired legs. Preoccupied with my own struggle, I hadn't noticed that Andrew was no longer running beside me. I turned to see his shrinking figure behind me. Eventually, he too dropped out, a victim of the hills. This was a surprise, as he had shown himself to be a strong distance runner. I carried on alone.

I reached the crest of a steep downhill on Spring Garden Road. Crossing a narrow bridge at the bottom of the hill brought me to the corresponding uphill. I knew this short but sharp incline marked the end of the hills, leaving me with only two miles to go to the finish. Perhaps fittingly for this point in the race, we ran by a large cemetery on York Boulevard, before cruising back into downtown Hamilton on a relatively easy, downhill stretch. I soldiered on to the finish, now a certainty. My time of 2:16 was poor, and I finished 116th. On unstable legs, I made my way back to the YMCA building that served as race headquarters. I retrieved my sweats and sat on the floor of the lobby to put them on. The building was crowded and humid and stinking of sweat and liniment. I looked around, proud of what I had done and content just to be part of this scene. I caught a glimpse of the winner, Dave Northey, a legend of road racing in Ontario. Even after my disappointing performance, I was hooked.

* * *

I continued to try other pursuits, but running soon occupied a prominent place in my life. For a while longer, I hung out with John, my best friend from the neighbourhood. We would often go to that same downtown YMCA to work out or swim or play basketball. In those days, the Y was a men's-only facility, with ancient weight equipment and a dingy pool, where scrawny old men shuffled back and forth across the deck.

John was, by that time, doing a lot of bodybuilding. We both admired a young phenomenon named Arnold Schwarzenegger, who was all over the magazines that John was fond of buying. John wanted to look like Arnold and dedicated himself to it. I preferred to lift lighter weights and do more reps, as that approach was more complementary to my athletics training.

My friend and I always got along well, even though we were quite different. We were in many ways, total opposites. I sensed that we were slowly drifting apart, but I still valued his company. He was utterly competitive and would turn everything—anything—into a competition. He would never quit until he had won. I enjoyed competing, but I also knew when I had had enough. Now, I wonder what I might have accomplished if I'd had even a fraction of John's competitive drive. The YMCA where we worked out had a tiny running track, with squared-off corners, where he would push me to run a mile as fast as I could. I was chuffed to realize that John had also accepted that I was becoming a runner. It was out of character for him to not even try to beat me at whatever it was we were doing.

Not only in sports was the distance growing between John and me. Our future paths were bound to diverge, because I knew my academic career would continue past high school. John was not a great student. He struggled to pay attention in school. On the other hand, I was an excellent student, committed and studious. I was curious about every subject, and I breezed through most of my classes. Like my friend, I sometimes had trouble paying attention, but for a different reason. I often found the proceedings to be a bit slow for my taste. I compensated by taking on a higher course load, which meant I could finish the five-year curriculum in four.

Given the ordeal that my older sister Kathleen had endured while fighting cancer, I was the first of my siblings to graduate and consider the question of what would come next. Fortunately, she recovered and started university the year after I did. In retrospect, I wonder if I missed an opportunity. I could have taken things at a slower pace and focused more on my growing passion for running.

As it was, I approached my imminent decision with almost complete ignorance. Mom had gone to vocational school and Dad had not even finished high school, so their ability to help me choose a career path was limited. They knew I was bright enough to go on to university, and they supported my doing so. It was a fortuitous meeting with a guidance counsellor that had a significant influence on the course of my life. He asked me some basic questions about what subjects I enjoyed the most. That was easy.

"Math and science, especially chemistry," I replied. I ventured a guess that that meant I should choose science as my course of study.

"Maybe. But given your marks, you might consider starting in engineering." He went on to explain that while the course load would be higher at first, if I decided after a year that I would like to switch to a science program, I could do it. Going the other way may not be feasible.

To a naïve kid like me, that made a lot of sense. At the time, I would have had difficulty explaining what an engineer did. It turned out to be one of the best decisions I ever made. By choosing engineering, I lit another flame. It was the first important, possibly life-changing, decision that I would take. And I had made the decision based not on rational analysis, but on a gut feel. It would not be the last time that I'd make an important decision that way.

While I prepared for post-secondary school, I was determined to make the most of my last year of high school athletics. My commitment to running was solid. I was passionate about the sport and totally absorbed with my training. The highlight of the year for me was the cross-country season. We won the senior boys' city championship and punched our ticket to the provincial championships in North Bay.

A small group of us made the long trek north for the season finale in November. We left Hamilton with high hopes. I don't remember much about the race itself, except for lots of mud, intimidating hills, and disappointing results for me and my teammates. We all struggled with the conditions. I was the first finisher of four from my school, and I was 134th overall. Despite our lack of impact on the race, we returned home satisfied with what we had achieved together. It was a great experience and one that further solidified the importance of running in my life.

Deb

AS THE WEEKS PASSED IN my last year of high school, I had whittled my choice of universities down to three, including two out-of-town schools. The idea of leaving home appealed to me, even though that would have meant a lot of planning. I had done none, and the time to decide was getting closer. Then, some welcome news arrived in the mail one day before the holidays. I had been offered an entrance scholarship to McMaster, a well-regarded university in my hometown. My decision had been made for me, given the advantages of living at home and more to the point, having my tuition fees covered.

Like many kids, I was totally bewildered by the first few weeks of university. Auditorium-sized classes were a whole new experience. It seemed that other students knew so much more about calculus and chemistry than I did. How would I survive this? Slowly, though, the fog lifted and gave way to a predictable routine. I reminded myself that hard work was something I had been dealing with for years. Besides, I was interested in all my subjects, and I was learning a lot. By Christmas, I was feeling more comfortable with the workload. And in the new year, I noticed that the classes seemed to have thinned out a little. There had been some early casualties. I was nowhere close to dropping out, so maybe I was cut out for this after all. Indeed, after an engaging discussion with my chemistry professor, he asked me if I would consider working as his lab assistant for the summer. I jumped at his offer.

My family was not known for overt displays of affection, but they were very much behind me. My Uncle John bought me a drafting desk so I would have a proper place to work. Then my Uncle Charlie gave me an HP-33C engineering calculator. Holding this magnificent machine in my hands, I was speechless. Whenever I turned it on, I felt accountable to my family to give my best effort. These may have been the nicest things anyone had ever done for me.

By my second year, I felt that I belonged at university. For those of us who had made it this far, it was time to split up into engineering disciplines. I had done well enough to earn my first choice, and it was easy—Chemical Engineering. In practical terms, that would mean that most classes from then on were small enough to be held in a room, rather than an auditorium. I picked up with my friends from first year, and began getting to know others, whom I would soon be spending a lot more time with. Everything seemed to be falling into place.

And the most important of the pieces fell into place when I met Deb.

It was in a class that we shared with other engineers. The subject was Statics and Dynamics. All engineers should know something about forces and centres of gravity, but for us chemical engineers this seemed to be a subject that would be of little practical use. We sat together at the back of the class. It was inevitable that there were a few testosterone-fuelled wisecracks from our group. I admit that I made my share. I could attribute our boorish antics to a feeling that by making it this far we had moved up on the campus pecking order. Whatever the reason, it was after I made what I considered to be a rather witty joke that an attractive, slim young woman with thick brown hair turned to me, with a look of disdain on her face.

"Gee, you're mouthy today, aren't you?" she said.

As she returned her gaze to the front of the classroom, I felt my face turn crimson. There were snorts of laughter from my friends and more than a few raised eyebrows.

I was instantly smitten. My head was spinning. Who was this girl?

I recovered enough after that first encounter to begin making enquiries, starting with a couple of fellow chemical engineers who seemed to know this girl well enough to sit with her regularly. Her name was Deborah Schlosser. She was from Toronto, and she lived in an apartment about a mile off campus.

After my less than auspicious start, I had some way to go to improve my standing with Deborah. It was not too hard to find opportunities for a few words with her from time to time. My initial impression was that she seemed smart and sophisticated, at least from my working-class perspective.

I figured that running might serve to show Deborah more about me. And coincidentally, I was getting more serious in that area. As I started my second year, I had decided to give athletics another try. That simply would not have been possible in first year. I went to the varsity cross-country tryouts, and I made the team. I was by no means a key member of the team, but that was beside the point. I was back into athletics, and I was part of a team for the time being.

The location of McMaster University, in the west end of Hamilton, is idyllic. The campus is adjacent to Cootes Paradise, a wetland area at the western tip of Lake Ontario. In Hamilton, the industrial heartland looms over the city, but from the vantage point of the university it is nothing more than a minor distraction. The trails and sports fields were as pleasant a place to run as I had ever seen. There was no better way to recharge after a long day of classes. I started to juggle my studies and the demands of varsity athletics.

Not that it was all pleasant, though. The field house was something out of a Dickens novel. The men's locker room was a dire spot in the basement of the Physical Education building. It was still the early days of the running boom, and equipment choices were less plentiful. For men, a jockstrap was still standard equipment. The routine was to go up to a counter and ask for a roll—that was a towel rolled up with a T-shirt and a jockstrap—from the attendant, usually a bored old guy who looked like he would rather be anywhere else. I cringed every time I handled the drab grey contents. Things usually improved once the running started.

My varsity running career was brief and unmemorable to anyone but me. I still get mail from McMaster to its athletic alumni, but that has always seemed a stretch. I did get a chance to try some prestigious track races, like the 5000-metre and the 3000-metre steeplechase. These were satisfying diversions, but it soon became clear that I would not be able to continue my balancing act much longer. One Friday afternoon, I cut short a midterm exam to catch a team bus that would take us to an out-of-town meet for the weekend. I left Hamilton knowing that I had done poorly on the exam because I had taken on too much. I was deluding myself.

As we drove to our destination, I sat staring out the window, realizing that the time had come for me to give this up. What was I thinking? I felt like a fool and a dismal failure. I thought about my brother, who by then was achieving national recognition as a high school track runner. Even if I didn't need to reach that level, and never could, all I had ever wanted was some of the same experiences. I was jealous of what he had. At the same time, I recognized where my own strengths lay. My priority had to be with academics, rather than athletics. I wondered whether athletics even had a place in my future.

Coming to my decision was the difficult part. I shed the burden of regimented training, and I was able to dedicate myself to my engineering studies. More than ever, I was convinced that I had made the right choice in pursuing this field of study. And to my surprise, I soon found another source of contentment with my decision. I realized that athletics did not have to be an all-or-nothing proposition for me. Instead, I worked out a comfortable arrangement, in which running was relegated to a secondary but still essential place in my life. For the next couple of years, I could look forward to running the trails and streets around the campus, strictly for relaxation. Once again, running was for fun, and I was in control.

One day, my feet seemed to have their own idea of where to go. I found myself running towards Deborah's building. Before I could stop myself, I was pushing the buzzer for her apartment. For a moment, I considered turning and running away.

"Hello," came her voice over the speaker. "Who is it?"

"It's Steve," I replied. I added, as an afterthought, "Steve Kelly."

A long pause.

"What do you want?"

That was a fair question, as up until that point I had not thought about it. I managed some excuse, perhaps that I was out for a run and needed a drink of water. Could she oblige? Reluctantly, she allowed me to come up. A bit of awkward chit-chat followed, with me no doubt making quite an impression as I dripped sweat in her doorway.

No one was more surprised than me when our relationship grew from that questionable start. I looked forward to sitting with Deborah—Deb—in class or in the library. Our common circle of friends made it easy for us to spend informal time together. Social events and class parties on the weekends were a chance to get to know each other better. She knew about jazz music and art and dance, and she made me want to know about them too. I was surprised that she was willing to tolerate my juvenile male interests. But it was strange that Led Zeppelin and Rush, and even the Boston Bruins, seemed to have lost their ability to hold my attention.

Before too long, Deb and I were an item. We have been together ever since.

* * *

My four years as an undergraduate student passed in the blink of an eye. As a small, close-knit group, we chemical engineers progressed through our third and fourth years, working with purpose and generally enjoying our time together. I formed close friendships with several of my classmates, while I barely knew others. It was a worthwhile experience to spend so much time together. We each contributed in our own way to the character of our class.

The question of what came after university started to come up in conversations. I worked another summer in the chemistry lab after my second year. However, my interest in the kind of close and intense work that was needed to make it as an academic had by then already waned. I needed a different experience.

I got what I asked for after my third year. I landed a summer job at Dofasco, working in the Environmental Control department, which is a busy group in a steel plant. Our offices were in portable work structures, in the shadow of the blast furnaces, deep in the heart of the sprawling plant site. What had been experienced at a safe distance as I grew up was now very real and very close. Nothing could have prepared me for the jarring assault on my senses.

I was assigned a demanding project. It required me to crawl around on top of the No. 1 Melt Shop, to measure the flow of gas in the exhaust ducting above a cauldron where liquid iron was converted into raw steel by blasting it with high pressure oxygen. Scrambling around the rafters inside the shop was terrifying—likely as close as one could get to the gates of hell. And from my vantage point on the roof, I could admire breathtaking views out over the lake as the soles of my work boots melted into its metal grating. I was being baked by two suns. One, the boiling liquid steel just below my feet, and the other, the familiar hot, humid sun of a Hamilton summer. Despite achieving modest success with my project, it was the end of my work in the steel industry. Where I would end up after graduation was still an open question.

I graduated in the spring of 1982 and immediately started working on my master's degree. My decision was more due to a precipitous downturn in the economy than it was to any burning desire to continue at school. Few of us got any kind of job in our field. I had been offered a novel project, one that would involve two of my favourite professors as my supervisors. They were teachers and mentors I had great respect for. My project would require me to split my time between Hamilton (for classes) and Sarnia (for field work). I would work in the Polysar plant, in Sarnia's Chemical Valley, with the objective of improving the reliability and control of a synthetic rubber manufacturing process.

I spent my first work term getting to know the technical team and the plant operators. Sarnia is a nice place to spend the summer. I had little to do in my spare time except run and play golf, so I did a lot of each. Deb, who had graduated with a degree in Chemistry, landed a job with Ontario Hydro, the provincial electrical utility, at a plant that produced heavy water for the province's nuclear reactors. She lived three hours' drive north of Sarnia, in a town called Port Elgin. We alternated driving back and forth between our two places, each in a new Honda Civic. Neither of us was ready to commit to living in the same location, due to the depressed job market.

* * *

My appreciation and love of athletics grew. I followed all the results for my latest heroes, the middle-distance stars Sebastian Coe and Eamonn Coghlan. Coe became a global sensation when he set three brilliant world records on the track, all within six weeks in the summer of 1979. But it was the *way* he ran, with elegance and effortless power—with passion—that I admired most.

Coghlan's specialty was the indoor mile. He had earned the nickname "Chairman of the Boards" due to his ability to perform well on tight, wooden indoor tracks. Deb humoured me for an evening in February 1981 at the Toronto Star Indoor Games, with its temporary track set up in Maple Leaf Gardens. I had run there as a schoolboy a few years earlier. We watched Coghlan win the mile in 3:55, an astounding achievement considering the quality of that track. I still have a black and white photograph that I snapped as he jogged around the track for his victory lap.

I can't be sure where I got the idea that I wanted to run a marathon. Maybe it was inevitable after running the Bay Race and reading about the exploits of Rodgers and Drayton. In the early 1980s, even as running continued to grow in popularity, the marathon was still mostly the domain of hard-core runners. Through my university years, I gained confidence with longer runs, and would often run more than ten miles in training. Basically, I think my curiosity got the better of me. All the reading I had done suggested that I should be able to run, if not race, the marathon.

I was uncoached, but I figured I knew enough about competitive running that I could comfortably develop my own training program. I found a training schedule that was endorsed by Brian Maxwell, a renowned Canadian marathoner. I liked it because it was simple. Maxwell called for a minimum of sixty miles per week leading up to the race, split out as follows: 5-5-10-5-10-5-20, with one or two sessions of speed work. I dove in. While I committed myself to the effort, the truth was that I rarely met the required weekly mileage, and I did almost no speed work. I followed the conventional wisdom of not running the full marathon race distance in training. So, the race itself would be the first time I attempted to run this far.

In theory, I could estimate my marathon performance from shorter races, as long as I did the work necessary to tackle the longer distance. At the time, I was running 10k races in the 37- to 39-minute range, which suggested a marathon time of between 2:50 and 3:00. That sounded alright to me, even though I had stretched the caveat about doing all the required training.

In 1982, the field of available races was paltry compared to today. Almost by default, I decided on the Toronto Marathon. It was becoming a major race on the Ontario calendar—by far the largest marathon—and it was close to home. Deb's parents lived in Toronto, so I would have a place to stay for the weekend. The early October schedule meant that race day weather could be just about anything. Heat and humidity were a real possibility, and for me that was the worst-case scenario.

As it turned out, the weather on race morning was agreeable. It was a fine late summer day, neither too hot nor too humid. I looked around at the start. I again found myself in a sea of road racing's hard men. And again, I wondered what I had signed up for. Apparently not much had changed when it came to the demographics of longer road races, even though by then the running boom was almost a decade old.

I was either inexperienced enough to assume that my preparations were adequate, or dumb enough to go ahead even if they were not. I set off at my target pace. I expected to see Deb a couple of times throughout the morning. Not being from Toronto, I did not really know what to expect out on the course. After the downtown start at Queen's Park, the route took us west, to some of the light industrial areas of Toronto. This section of the course was exposed and tedious. Not unusual for road races at the time, water stations were infrequent. I passed the half marathon mark in about 1:25, which put me in my target range, at least mathematically. I was feeling reasonably good. About twenty minutes later, I had a fleeting thought, which began a downward spiral of my confidence.

I've gone a long way—sixteen miles—but that still leaves ten miles to go.

Here was the first chink in my armour. It was the beginning of the end. I felt my pace slowing for the next few miles. While I was undeniably making forward progress, I could not get the negative thoughts out of my head. Then I started noticing blisters and other discomforts. I walked for the first time before I had reached twenty miles. Then I walked again. And again. For a while, I could convince myself to start jogging again, but eventually, even that became harder. Was this "the wall" I had read about, the mythical point beyond twenty miles when the body's glycogen stores were depleted, and the body resorted—unwillingly—to burning fat for fuel?

I knew Deb and her parents would be waiting for me on Lake Shore Boulevard, not far from their family home. I was already in bad shape when I saw them, and I still had about five miles to go. It was torture to get my legs moving at anything more than a walking pace.

After what seemed like an eternity, I reached University Avenue and began the last stretch north, to the finish on the track at Varsity Stadium. I was reduced to walking a block and then jogging a couple. Scores of runners passed me. Within the last mile, I was determined to see this through to the finish, even with my hopes of a decent performance stranded somewhere behind me on Lake Shore Boulevard. Now inside the stadium, I managed a feeble and totally unnecessary finishing sprint. What difference did it make at that stage?

I crossed the line in 3:15:24, in 621st place. There were 1,871 official finishers that day.

I was totally demoralized. The marathon had defeated me. I

thought it would take me a while to get over that experience. It helped that I had just begun my first semester of graduate classes—I was swamped. Even so, running remained an important part of my routine. In fact, in that period running was one of the things that kept me sane. One of my professors, Dr. Taylor, was a novice runner, and we occasionally went out for a jog together. We often discussed training techniques and he expressed his interest in tackling the marathon. He was intrigued by the theoretical aspects of distance running. For my part, I eagerly shared all my learning, which was based on a small dataset of one poorly executed race.

When I returned to Sarnia for another summer work term, I again found myself with a lot of free time in the evenings and weekends. I dedicated myself to improving on my poor performance in last fall's marathon. It was during this summer that I pushed my mileage to levels I had never reached before. My peak weekly total was over ninety miles. I had a five-mile circuit that I ran often, and it was not uncommon for me to run three laps—fifteen miles—on a weeknight. I would get up early on the weekends and run out of town along Lakeshore Road, going well past the next town, Bright's Grove, before turning around.

By then I had found a compatible group of runners that was affiliated with the downtown Y in Sarnia. Some of my co-workers at Polysar were committed runners, and we often trained together. A talented local runner, Will Burris, led our fledgling group.

I decided to try a rematch with the Toronto Marathon. But before the race there was another Sarnia summer to enjoy. I spent a lot of time with my thesis supervisor, Dr. Hoffman, as he and his wife seemed happy to take me under their wing. He and I would often play nine holes of golf in the evenings. I was invited to many meals at the Hoffman house, which was ideally situated on Lake Huron. Deb and I continued to commute back and forth for weekend visits. It was a blissful summer, centred on work, play and of course, running.

All good things do come to an end, and in late August I returned to Hamilton for another couple of semesters. I would finish up my course work, and with any luck, complete my thesis. The job market was still miserable, so my future remained uncertain. Worse, I was tiring of my project. I had come to see the downside of having two supervisors, as it began to feel like I was preparing not one, but two, thesis reports.

As I grappled with this burden, I was consoled by returning to the comfortable lifestyle of a graduate student. Being back at McMaster meant I could once again run in Cootes Paradise. It was more than an ever-present diversion. It was a place of solace when I felt unequal to the tasks before me. How I treasured those peaceful, mind-clearing runs!

I began to realize that this was an essential part of the learning process, particularly if a thorny problem was weighing me down. Although I may have set my mind to think through the problem while I ran, it was more likely that my mind would find its own path, just as I took my own turns on the trails or the streets. Whatever the process, which I could appreciate if not fully understand, I inevitably saw things more clearly after returning to work.

Before I got too deeply into academic pursuits, there was the small matter of a marathon to run. I felt better prepared for the 1983 race than I had a year earlier. I had focused my training over the summer to add more mileage. I redoubled my efforts to research and implement the prevailing theories of training, which for the lone runner were found mostly in magazine articles and a few reference books. I was thankful for my many discussions with Dr. Taylor, whose enthusiasm for running as a research project had not waned.

I arrived at the start line feeling slightly less intimidated amid the hard men, but when it was over the result was more or less the same. I managed to hold off the collapse better than I had in 1982, but my death march up University Avenue was almost identical. I limped home in just under 3:10 and finished in 421st position. I had shaved six minutes off my time, but I was even less pleased with my performance. The puzzle of the marathon remained unsolved and would have to remain so for the time being.

Yes, That's the Edmonton in Alberta

AS MY THESIS PROJECT CREPT towards its conclusion, there were big decisions to make. First among these was the question of where Deb and I would live and work. We got engaged in 1983, and the prospect of staying apart for work reasons was not very appealing to either of us. She was still working at the heavy water plant. I had no assurance that a job would be forthcoming at Polysar, even though I had worked for them, on and off, for almost two years. The economy remained weak, and this was a hurdle when it came to their deciding whether to hire me. They eventually scrabbled together a job offer, but it was for the best that I ended up not working there.

I did return to Sarnia for the summer of 1984, this time with a different employer. As luck would have it, one of my instructors at McMaster was an adjunct professor whose full-time job was with Shell Canada. He arranged an interview, and that led to a job offer in their Sarnia Refinery. Steve would be my first supervisor, even though he worked in Toronto, at Shell's head office. He specialized in using computers to control industrial processes, which was a novel concept in the mid-1980s. My thesis stood me in good stead for that type of work. Steve and I had hit it off when I first met him, so the prospect of joining him at Shell made sense to both of us. It seemed like an achievement to have even landed a job offer in those difficult times.

For this, my third and last stint in Sarnia, I shared a house with two of my engineering classmates. I continued to train, and train with conviction. I was still involved with the runners from the Sarnia Y. I spent a lot of time in the evenings and weekends on short and medium runs, and I devoted the weekends to the long runs that were a core part of my training program. Will Burris had added a weekly interval session for our Y running group. Through the spring and summer, I felt my fitness improving, as I adapted and honed my previous training ideas.

I began to feel like this would be my turn to deliver a worthy marathon performance in Toronto, on the assumption that I would run it again in the fall. All the elements were in my training program. But it was not to be. Deb and I set our wedding date for early September, which effectively shelved the idea of a fall marathon. For a time, I kidded her that it was her fault I never reached my potential in the marathon.

Although our longer-term future was still up in the air, things were about to get a little more complicated for Deb and me. We had not yet answered the open question of where we would live and how we would align our careers. One day in the spring, as I was wrapping up my project and preparing to leave the university, Steve dropped by my office. He was not a shy person, and without wasting time, he let me know that Shell's plans for me did not involve staying in Sarnia, as I had been led to believe. Rather, they wanted to move me to a new refinery they would soon be starting up in Edmonton. That was the Edmonton in Alberta, a world away from everything I knew.

I was meeting Deb that weekend, and I had to think carefully about how to share this news. When we were together, I steered the conversation to the question of our plans. I snuck up on the main question.

"If you could live anywhere in Canada, where would it be?" I asked.

"I think I'd eventually like to live in Toronto," she replied. Spoken like a Toronto girl.

"What about Alberta? Do you think you would ever want to live there?"

"Oh, no. I'd hate to live in Calgary," she said.

I had to play my one remaining card. "And what about Edmonton?" I cringed for the answer.

"That would be even worse!"

"You aren't making this any easier. I have something to tell you."

"What's that?" she asked. Suspicion was written all over her face.

"Shell wants to move us to Edmonton. The job they offered me is at their new refinery."

She sat for what seemed like an eternity, even though it was probably only about thirty seconds. I waited in silence.

"Okay, let's try it. But we should come back to Ontario after a year or two."

Of all the answers I thought I might get, this was probably the best one I could have hoped for. In fact, it was a totally sensible suggestion.

I thought I had better make sure we were both on the same page. "Are you sure you'd be okay moving to Edmonton?"

"Yeah, let's do it. But I don't want to live there permanently."

At that moment, I had even more proof that I had made the best possible decision asking this woman to marry me. We toasted our prospects and looked ahead to a new adventure together. At the time, we knew absolutely nothing about Edmonton or Alberta.

* * *

We were married in September 1984 in Toronto in a modest ceremony. We had a chance to visit Edmonton before moving there. In late October, we left from Toronto for a house-hunting trip. The temperatures on that day were +22 degrees Celsius in Toronto and -22 degrees Celsius in Edmonton. It was a rather rude introduction to the city. A day later, as we drove north on Ninety-seventh Street in a howling whiteout, we were both thinking the same thing.

"Where the heck are we moving to, Siberia?" Deb asked.

We connected with a real estate agent who would later help us find a home in the neighbourhood we had decided on. That was not a simple process, and with us it rarely is. One thing I learned early on in our life together is that Deb has an uncanny ability to navigate a new city and find a neighbourhood that meets our needs. It does not always make finding a home easy, but it has served us well. In the meantime, we signed a lease on an apartment in the northeast of the city.

Our move to Edmonton took place a few weeks later, in December 1984. We had ventured into the great unknown with our arrival in Edmonton. It was the beginning of our long connection to Alberta.

* * *

Not all the developments were happy during this period. I consider it more than a small miracle that my siblings and I all dodged a bullet as we passed adolescence and became young adults. That bullet was alcoholism. Surrounded as we were by several alcoholics, it is unclear how we all managed to avoid the curse. I have a couple of theories to explain it. I have not spoken to my siblings about it, and they may have their own explanations. Maybe it doesn't even matter, as long as it just is.

My father, his father and two of his brothers were alcoholics, and yet none of us followed the same path. That is mainly due to Mom's positive influence. We all benefited from the protective environment that Mom created and tried to maintain as we grew up. My siblings each had their own positive influences, career paths, hobbies, and other interests that offered satisfying counterarguments to alcohol's attractions. I am forever grateful for that.

The other factor that is certainly true in my case, and really the point of even dwelling on this part of my story, is the positive influence that running had in shaping my personality. I will never know what Dad was searching for, or why he thought he would find it at the bottom of a bottle. Maybe he was trying to fill a gap in his own life. Perhaps alcohol helped make Dad the person he wanted to be. Or as I theorized, it may have been his way to deal with the deep worry he felt for my sister Kathleen. Whatever the reason, it was a shame because he was actually a special character—charismatic, witty, and smart.

* * *

This is a good point for me to say a little more about Kathleen. She survived her two-year nightmare of cancer treatments as a teenager, and another round of treatments a few years later when the disease re-asserted itself. Only years after that did I learn how long the odds really were against her. I had been seated next to a friend of a friend at a large holiday dinner. She was a pediatrician. Over dinner, we talked about our families and our careers. When she told me about her work, I volunteered a comment about Kathleen and her childhood cancer diagnosis. My dinner partner was interested, and she asked if I recalled any of the details of my sister's illness.

"Yes, I do. Kathleen had Ewing's sarcoma. She had a tumour on her collarbone." I replied.

"And did she… survive?" Christine asked, hesitating as if she already knew the answer.

"Yes, she did. She's alive and well and living with her husband in Ontario."

After a long pause, Christine said something that has stuck with me ever since.

"I'm so glad to hear that. You see, I've had the unenviable task of telling the parents of children who have the same terrible diagnosis as your sister, that their child has a chance of beating the disease. It's just that I've never personally known of a case where this has actually happened. Now, when I'm telling these other parents, I will at least I be able to think about your sister and know that she *did* beat the odds. Thank you so much for sharing your story."

Christine confirmed what I've always known—that my sister Kathleen is a miracle.

* * *

As a young adult, I did not know that running had headed off my need to go through a similar search as my father. I do now. That void, if it existed at all, was neatly—in fact, ideally—filled by an activity that cleared my mind, shaped my body and nourished my spirit better than any alcoholic drink I know of. Running was an ideal drug, and it became my addiction, even if I would not have been able to see things in those black and white terms at the time.

I need to continue the story of Dad's challenges with alcohol, though, as difficult as that is to do. The consequences of his drinking were long-term and profound. I considered myself somewhat fortunate because I was out of the house and on my own before my siblings. I knew Dad was spiralling down. More than once on my visits home, I found him in the basement drinking on his own, simply chugging a bottle. We would exchange knowing glances. He was aware that we were all wise to his self-destructive behaviour. My mother could recite a list of the many small tricks he used to try and hide his drinking. What she or any of us could have done about it, I'm not sure.

His addiction came close to tearing my parents apart, as we reached our early twenties. Mom internalized the pain and suffering, and eventually assumed the complete burden of holding the family together. And she did that while trying with all the tools at her disposal to get Dad to stop drinking. She sought outside help, which was intended for the loved ones of an alcoholic more than the person responsible. I think she eventually came to accept that the problem was his, not hers. As far as addressing the root cause, that was a futile effort. If anything, as the years dragged on, and as we all moved away from home, our departure seemed to exacerbate the problems at home.

* * *

We were alone in a new city, with me worrying about my new job and Deb worrying about finding one. Our first year in Edmonton was extremely hard on her. Living as a couple for the first time, it was just as hard on our relationship. It did not help that the winter of 1984–1985 was particularly harsh, even by Alberta standards. We were living in a small apartment outside of the downtown core, and we felt truly isolated. Deb is a proud and independent person, used to looking after herself. This was not the life she had envisioned. At least I had the benefit of seeing other people at the refinery during the work week. Even so, the plant was about fifty kilometres northeast of the city. Over the long winter, as I made my daily drive to and from the plant in the dark, it felt like we had indeed moved to Siberia.

With a concerted effort, I finished my master's thesis, and I returned to Hamilton in the spring of 1985 to defend it. Deb started perusing the job ads, at first with little success. Eventually, she landed a job as a research assistant at the Cross Cancer Institute, which helped ease her anxiety about our move. It would not be the last significant career change she would make. She never totally warmed up to the city, but her work as a cancer research scientist did turn into a positive and satisfying experience. I was very proud of her.

We started to branch out a little. Gradually, we were able to reach a kind of equilibrium with Edmonton. We discovered the city's lively cultural and restaurant scene. We made friends through our work and started spending time with them socially. And we learned that Edmonton's lush river valley was a spectacular location for walking, cross-country skiing, or running.

In 1986, we bought our first home, two blocks north of the river, in a neighbourhood called Highlands. The house was old and quirky, with sloping floors, but it was comfortable. It sat on a large lot with a variety of apple trees. We became close with the neighbours in the house behind us. They owned a restaurant in the city. We reached an easy bargain with them—they could help themselves to any fruit on our property, if we could share in the baking that resulted from it.

I joined the Edmonton Roadrunners, an active local club. Later, I assumed the role of newsletter editor and took a few turns as race director. It was a good group, with a large contingent of talented runners. Long runs on Sunday were ideal for making new friends. The racing scene was busy, with quality races and strong competition. Our club organized a series of 5k races over the winter months that went ahead regardless of the weather. I continued to make progress as a competitive runner, recording some worthy results in the 5- and 10-milers that were still popular race distances. Ten miles became my favourite race distance, and it may always be.

I took another shot at the marathon in 1986. Edmonton had a somewhat erratic history relating to marathons, but for a couple of years there was an iteration that started and finished near our house. I signed up, perhaps counting more on a carryover of my decent fitness from 1984 than on anything I had done since then. I regularly did runs of two hours or a bit more, still using Maxwell's "5-5-10-5-10-5-20" mileage program. This was an exceptional way to explore the river valley pathway system. Going into the race, I knew I was short of the mileage I really needed, and I was still not doing any speed work. Despite these shortcomings in my training, in a small field, on a warm day, I ran a race that I could almost be happy with. I finished nineteenth in 3:01, which was a personal best—a PB—by eight minutes. I felt much better in the closing miles than I had in both my previous marathon attempts. Maybe I was getting the hang of this.

We ventured out from Edmonton to explore the sights around central Alberta. We made our first trips to the mountains—Jasper and Banff—in our under-powered Honda Civics. We fell for the magnificence of the Rockies and returned often. I snapped a lot of photos with my trusty manual Canon camera, doing my best to emulate another of my heroes, the great landscape photographer Ansel Adams. We drove east of the city to the little gem that was Elk Island National Park, and visited small towns dotted all around Edmonton. Trips to Calgary, to connect with our school friends Lisa and John, led us to realize that it was a city more to our liking than Edmonton. We had nothing against Edmonton, as such, but I think it was the isolation that we felt most keenly.

In May 1987, we made a trip to Calgary so I could take yet another turn at the marathon. The Calgary Marathon was a large and well-established race in Alberta. And this time, I had put in the miles, in the river valley and on the quiet country roads around the refinery. I had run in the long spring evenings that Edmonton's northerly latitude provided. I felt ready for a breakthrough, and it came. I shaved another few minutes off my PB, running 2:58 and finishing forty-second overall. A picture taken at the finish line shows me looking skyward, as if to say, "Thank God!" It felt as if a large weight had been lifted from my shoulders. After four attempts in five years, I experienced the joy and satisfaction that came with being a sub-three-hour marathoner!

January 1988 marked an even better milestone. We welcomed our son Matthew into our lives. Matthew was a gentle, intelligent child. He surprised us when he was about eighteen months old, by silently pointing out all the letters in the alphabet. He was reading everything shortly afterwards. He would grow up a shy, quiet kid, who was seemingly more content to observe than to participate. Now, he is a worldly young man, fiercely independent and confident in his own abilities. He makes us immensely proud.

* * *

The Jasper–Banff Relay Race was put on by the Chasquis Running Club in Edmonton. Unlike a lot of other races at that time, Chasquis events were consistently well organized. And for years, their mountain relay was the jewel in the Alberta race calendar. The Chasquis relay ran from 1980 through 2000, and it was re-launched by another group years later. In its original format, which I think many veteran runners would say they prefer, the relay started in Jasper at noon on the first Saturday in June and progressed from north to south until the teams reached Banff. The course was 284 kilometres long and was divided into stages of varying degrees of difficulty.

It was a monumental event. Imagine 120 teams of seventeen runners, when the relay was at its peak. Just getting that many people to Jasper for the start required a major effort. Now, imagine all the support teams and vehicles and volunteers, grinding their way down the highway, like in some kind of precision military exercise, through the day and night and next morning, in all kinds of weather, through some of the most breathtaking scenery in the world. But best of all, imagine experiencing this majestic scenery in the open air, quietly running down the highway, rather than seeing it speed by your car window.

The relay was already hugely popular in 1988, when I signed up to run on a Roadrunners mixed team. My club often had two or three teams entered in the race. Our team's goal was simple—we intended to win our division. We had a strong team of five women and twelve men. One of our female runners would later go on to become a triathlon world champion.

I knew little of what was to come, just what I had heard from my teammates. I considered myself a veteran, but this event was unlike anything I had done before. Our early runners put us into a competitive position, even vying for the overall race lead. I tried to keep myself calm through the day. That was difficult to do in such a picturesque setting and with a team that was putting in a great collective effort. Our runners kept us in contention through the race's strenuous climbs, Stage 6 to the Columbia Icefields and Stages 10 and 11 to Bow Summit, the highest point on the route. The impressive views were matched by our team's gutsy performances.

I helped out by supporting our runners on the road, keeping in mind that I needed to conserve energy for what was coming soon. My nerves increased as the relay ground on through the long afternoon and evening of early June. Darkness gradually took hold, increasing the tension even further. I was assigned to Stage 13, meaning that I would not even begin running until about 1 A.M. This was not something I had practised. The night was moonless. How would I handle running in the total darkness of a mountain park? The cumulative effort, the slow drip of energy, required to support my teammates over many hours was taking its toll, but sleep was out of the question. I had to make do with a bit of fitful rest in one of the support vehicles.

At midnight, I was dropped off at the Mosquito Creek

campground, the exchange point marking the start of my leg. I had studied the race profile. I knew that at twenty kilometres, Stage 13 was the longest in the relay. It was also steeply downhill for much of its length. While I was not a particular specialist in downhill running, that did not seem to be a major issue. It would prove to be the least of my worries.

As I checked in, a race official told me that a grizzly bear warning had been issued for my stage. What had he just said? I tried to stay calm. My pre-race stretching and jogging routine at the exchange point may have eased my nerves a little, but the prospect of encountering a grizzly in the pitch dark was less than appealing.

My appointed time to run was approaching. The usual practice at the mountain relays is to have a spotter read out team numbers as runners pass the one-mile-to-go point in the previous stage. After what seemed an eternity, I heard the radio call out team number 39. I made my last-minute preparations.

The protocol for dealing with a bear was to have team support vehicles make prescribed stops along the course, so that runners would never be more than a mile back down the road from their vehicle. Some comfort, I thought, if the bear were to grab me somewhere in between.

I took the handoff from my teammate, Bob, and plunged into the void. Just then, a crack of thunder announced the arrival of an unusual nighttime thunderstorm. I must be cursed, I thought. If I believed in bad luck, Stage 13 was providing proof of it that night. I headed away from the shelter of the exchange point. Within seconds, I was drenched.

I promptly learned a few lessons about overnight stages in the Jasper–Banff Relay. First, and not surprisingly, it can be dark in the mountains. I had no headlamp, so I had to rely on the light from a glow-stick I held in my right hand. That tiny source of light, reflected from the white painted line on the side of the highway, was worthless against the pounding rain. Making things worse was the glare of the headlights from oncoming cars. I had to avert my eyes to preserve whatever vision I had. I was truly running blind.

The first mile was a harrowing experience, and the sight of my support vehicle could not have been more welcome. My teammates went to great lengths to make sure I was fine before they headed off down the road. Perhaps sensing my growing panic, they offered to stop more frequently. I readily agreed, and I soon realized that the sight of our team vehicle, which I could make out from a long distance, was going to be key to my success on this night. Its taillights were like a lighthouse, guiding me through this stormy sea. And although I literally was in a storm, once I was soaked it made little difference that the rain continued to fall.

My mind began playing tricks on me. My senses were in overdrive, given the bear warning and other distractions. Gurgling noises from little creeks next to the road caused me to jump, and I started seeing bear-shaped shadows being thrown up by car headlights.

I took stock of my situation. I was running reasonably well, all things considered. The rain began to ease up. It would soon stop, leaving me to finish the stage in relative comfort. Given that we were well into the race, this was now an individual time trial. I had one task now—push the pace. I knew I was far from the slowest runner in the race, so it was with some surprise that I heard footsteps of a runner, and not a bear, behind me. There had been no one behind me earlier, at least I didn't think so. Had the rain drowned out the sound? No, no, the sound of footsteps was definitely getting louder as this runner gained on me. I tried to pick up my pace, but to no avail. The mystery runner pulled up beside me. I glanced over at him in the darkness.

"Chris! How are you doing?"

I was shocked to see that it was a fellow that I had known and competed against in high school. I had not seen him at the exchange point, but it was the middle of the night, after all.

"Hi Steve," he said. "I'm doing fine. How about you?"

I mumbled something about this crazy stage, which had just gotten even stranger. I mean, what were the odds of "running into" someone I last saw about ten years earlier, out here in almost exactly the middle of nowhere?

We chatted for a minute. I learned from Chris that he was living in Calgary, and that he was running for his corporate team. With relief, I recalled from our high school days that he was a stronger runner than me. He had been a city champion several times over. Resistance was apparently futile, so I wished him well as he pushed past me. Our individual time trials ground on.

The end of my unbelievable run was near. After more than an hour on the road, the support arrangements with my teammates in the van were well-rehearsed. The rain had let up. I was even getting used to the pitch blackness. I noticed that all the downhill running had begun to affect my gait. After all I had been through, the last thing I needed was to trip, so I focused on the ground I could see in front of me and made sure to lift my feet. I cruised into the exchange area for Stage 14 and made the handoff to our next runner, Sheila, without further incident.

We fought off our collective fatigue through a misty dawn by cheering ourselves hoarse for our last three runners and by helping rescue another team when their van needed a boost. We went on to finish second in the mixed division, losing out by 34 minutes to an American team, after an epic nineteen-hour battle. As a small consolation, we broke the previous mixed team record, and we finished fifteenth overall in a strong field. Our success was mainly due to standout performances by our women runners. I had certainly held my own and poured every ounce of my energy into supporting my teammates. I had even added my own memorable story to this already storied event. Was I ever spent after that weekend! The drive back to Edmonton seemed interminable.

* * *

I would go on to run the Jasper–Banff Relay several more times, on teams that generally did quite well. And I ran in the other multi-stage mountain relays that began to spring up. I have already mentioned the K–100 Relay. It was first contested in 1986 and has been a staple on the Alberta race calendar for years. According to my somewhat sketchy records, I've run that race six times, going back to its earliest days. There was even a Banff–Calgary Relay for a few years.

Running in the mountain relays can be an exhilarating experience, and I thrived in the atmosphere of a competitive team. That said, running on such a team meant making a huge commitment. I would throw myself completely into the enterprise. There was something about the lure of the unknown—the realization that no matter how much planning we did, we could never anticipate everything that might happen on race day. I certainly learned first-hand some of those lessons on that dark, stormy night along the Icefields Parkway.

As for the mountain relay format, I always found individual time trials to be challenging to run. (It was even tougher in the days before we had GPS watches to give us instant pacing feedback.) I never wanted to let my teammates down, so I sometimes took off too fast, only to pay the price later. I know that a well-executed relay stage is a performance one can be proud of.

It seemed that no subsequent relay could ever compare with my first Jasper–Banff race experience. Maybe it was because I had invested so much in the 1988 race and got so much in return. If only for a few days, it had managed to rekindle my best memories of taking up running and learning what it meant to truly be part of a team. To be part of something bigger than myself. For me, that Edmonton Roadrunners mixed team crystalized everything positive about competitive running: total commitment, both to my individual performance and in support of my teammates; thrilling competition, lasting the better part of a day; and a uniquely Canadian event in the mountain parks. One look at my medal from that race still evokes a flood of positive feelings.

Running Streaks ... And Strokes

IT WAS EARLY JULY 2017. I was well into a running streak that I had started on December 1, 2012. To keep the streak going, I had to run at least one mile every day. Starting a streak was an unusual thing for me to have done, since I had never bought into the idea that runners, even dedicated competitive runners like me, needed to run every day. My approach to training had evolved into a pattern of several key workouts each week and a long run on the weekend. Other days were, by definition, easy days, which usually included running but may just as likely have been days off. So for me, the whole idea of a running streak made little sense.

That said, I appreciate what it takes to carry on a running streak. I have known a number of streakers through the years. This evolutionary branch of the running population is an eccentric lot. Most serious runners of the last few decades would have heard of Ron Hill, the great British marathoner and Olympian, whose 52-year streak—which ended in 2017—is legendary. To running streakers, Ron Hill is a patron saint, a person who is universally admired and spoken of with great reverence. He died in 2021.

I've mentioned Will Burris, a running mentor and occasional

coach in Sarnia during my work stints there. In addition to being a fine runner, Will had some kind of long streak going, the details of which escape me. What I do remember is a story he told us, of how he continued his streak through a vasectomy. Without intending the pun, I'd say that took balls.

The streakers I knew best were my brother Paul and my good friend in Calgary, Rob. While Paul and Rob were far short of Ron Hill, they had each managed to compile impressive streaks. Rob would entertain me with heroic stories of the close calls he had overcome to keep his streak going. Rob and Paul were both talented runners, so I was keen to get them together when Paul and his wife Shelley visited us in Calgary. In an amazing coincidence, Paul and Rob had started their streaks within a week of each other, going back to January 1980.

We decided to do a long run starting from Rob's house. He lived near Fish Creek Park, a large park south of the city. I had run there many times, but I did not know the trails and the routes very well. Instead, I counted on my running partners to direct me. Our outing did not turn out well for me, as Rob and Paul instantly bonded, having in common their almost identical streaks and their prodigious running abilities. They put it into another gear and ditched me halfway through our run, leaving me bewildered on my solo return to Rob's house.

But back to my own running streak. I had been feeling a bit adrift and unmotivated in late 2012. As had happened occasionally in my running career, I lacked direction and a goal. I felt like I was going through the motions. During a visit to our local running store, Strides, I learned that they were promoting a December Running Streak. It was billed as a way of giving people a worthwhile goal—run at least a mile a day—over the holidays. On a whim, I signed up. It was just what I needed. I cruised through December and kept on going.

My streak grew to months, and then years. Admittedly, there were many days when I felt chained to this thing I had created, and that I was once again going through the motions. Maybe I was looking to collect a few close calls of my own, as I worked to keep my streak going. And I did. Several months after I started, I had to plan my daily runs around a colonoscopy. I was once reduced to running back and forth in a motel room on a rainy night in Norman Wells, Northwest Territories. However, because it was only a minimum of a mile per day, I felt that I could keep the streak going indefinitely. In fact, I had been talking to a work colleague about it in June 2017, and I said something like "it'll be five years on December 1, which is a sure thing."

Famous last words.

* * *

On July 4, a couple of days after our ill-fated long run, Mahedi and I met up again at Edworthy. This time, we would tackle an interval workout. After a warm-up, we planned to do three repeats of 2k at our 10k race pace, with a 1k slow jog in between. I was understandably reluctant after my difficulties a couple of days earlier. But on this day, Mahedi and I had curiously switched places. This time, he was struggling, and I felt quite normal. Mahedi and I were so in tune that I did not even have to glance over. I knew he had fallen off the pace before the end of our first 2k repeat. We did our recovery jog together, so I could check that he was okay. He waved me on, and I ran the remaining intervals on my own.

Later, as we reconvened in the parking lot, he admitted that this had just not been his day. He had bailed out on the 2k repeats, but he did manage to do several shorter intervals, effectively salvaging the workout. We agreed that it was a smart move on his part. We did a brief cooldown jog together, laughed at the change in our circumstances, and made plans to meet up again soon.

Then my world changed.

I woke up for what I expected would be a normal workday on July 5, with a strange sensation in my left arm and leg. I may have had the same feeling a few hours earlier when I got out of bed to go to the bathroom, but I can't be sure. I recalled feeling unsteady, groggy, not quite myself. In the morning, I felt something like the "pins and needles" sensation that comes from sleeping wrong. But this was different, more of a heavy and weak feeling, and both limbs were affected. My leg felt clumsy, and I had trouble getting down the stairs.

I skipped my breakfast and sat for a few minutes, thinking. Wait, wasn't there some kind of mnemonic? A word to check symptoms. But it couldn't be *that*. I know, I'll look at myself in the mirror. There was the same old mug staring back at me. I tried moving my limbs, and they responded. They just didn't feel right.

I decided that I should mention this to Deb, so I awkwardly made my way back upstairs and woke her. We talked. I *could* talk. That was another check. And she confirmed that I looked normal. Still, I felt odd enough that we agreed a call to 911 made sense.

Minutes later, we heard an ambulance approaching. By then, the feeling had largely passed. But they were already at the door, three of them, coming inside. I sat in my front hall chair, answering the EMS technicians' questions while they checked my vital signs. Since I was already feeling better, I proposed that we just forget the whole affair. I apologized for wasting their time. They assured me that this was not a concern, that they saw this sort of thing often, and that calling 911 was the right thing to have done. Apparently, they were not going to let me call this off.

I overheard the lead technician conferring with Deb, about

where they were planning to take me. I learned quickly what the main considerations were for this decision.

"Maybe we should go to the Rockyview Hospital. It's closer, and besides, the parking is better," Deb said. She had always been a practical person.

The EMS lead proposed taking me to the Foothills Medical Centre instead.

"If he's had a *stroke*, he'll end up there anyway," he said.

"Did he say *stroke*?" I asked myself. The word hit me like a gut punch.

With the initial checks done and an IV needle taped to my arm, I walked to the ambulance, unaided. I chatted with the technicians during the short ride to the Foothills emergency room. Deb and I sat a long time in the ER waiting room and then in an examination area. We talked to a young doctor about my symptoms and he ordered a CT scan on my head and neck.

Deb and I decided that she should go home. She had a few other things to do that day, and there was no reason for her to sit there with me. She left me with a bottle of water and some snacks. We agreed that I would call her later to pick me up.

After an uncomfortable wait of several hours, the same doctor came over to me and explained what they had found in the scan. I don't know what I expected to hear, but what he told me was shocking. He explained that I had a near blockage of one of the major arteries into my brain. In medical jargon, it was a "proximal near occlusion of the left vertebral artery." I had never heard of a vertebral artery, and I wasn't hearing much of what he told me in any event.

I was sent home with a clinical report and prescriptions for aspirin and Plavix, two drugs which would prevent platelets from sticking to plaque in my arteries. I was told that I should expect a call from the Foothills Stroke Prevention Clinic, and that I should get together with them as soon as possible. Deb picked me up, and as I sat in the car on the way home, stunned, all I could think was *How is this possible?* I read and re-read the clinical report, and even though I didn't understand the terminology, I knew it did not sound good.

One thing I made sure to check before leaving the ER was that I could continue to run. To my surprise, I was assured that I could, but that I should take it easy and not do any strenuous workouts.

* * *

July 5 was a Wednesday. I spent an anxious day or two, trying to make sense of what I had heard. As luck would have it, I had my phone on silent mode when the stroke clinic called me that Friday. I only picked up their call late in the afternoon. Their message said that I should call them back, but by the time I did so they had already closed for the week.

I stayed close to home over the weekend, working on small jobs around the house and editing a lengthy report that was due a few days later. Although these tasks took my mind away from worrying about what was going on with my plumbing, it was not a relaxing weekend.

I got to the office at my regular time on Monday and called the stroke clinic as soon as they were open.

"Oh, Mr. Kelly. Just a moment—" the nurse said.

After a pause, she asked, "Could you come in this afternoon?" It was not really a question.

"Sure," I replied, with trepidation in my voice.

I rearranged my schedule and took a cab to the hospital. I met one of the clinic nurses, and then a young resident. He explained the anatomy of the head and neck, and what last week's CT scan had shown them. He spoke in terms I could understand—after all, it is liquid flow in pipes, something familiar to a chemical engineer.

Then he drew me a sketch of the typical arterial configuration and pointed out the carotids and the vertebrals. He showed me the location of the proximal occlusion of my left vertebral artery. Finally, he explained what a stoke is and why it is so important to take action when a transient ischemic attack—a TIA—occurs. *Ischemic* refers to a restriction in blood flow. When blood flow to the brain is temporarily interrupted, it causes stroke symptoms. This may only last a short time, and that's why TIAs are often called mini-strokes. The concern is that they may signal the onset of a more serious stroke.

Before I left the clinic I met the lead clinician, Dr. Phil Barber. The topic of our discussion was stroke prevention. I took from this that I had perhaps not had an actual stroke. Rather, it seemed that my symptoms of the last month or more were still being interpreted as warning signs by the doctors. In other words, we were now going to try to prevent a catastrophic event. Dr. Barber wrote me prescriptions for Lipitor (a cholesterol-lowering statin) and more Plavix.

I admit that I got a bit impatient as the meetings went on. Everyone in the clinic seemed more interested in signing me up for a large study they were conducting than in dealing with my specific issue. I understood that by signing up for the study, I would gain faster access to an MRI, so I grudgingly agreed. By doing so, I also gave my consent to some follow-up tests. The key point was that I left the clinic with an appointment for an MRI on the following day, Tuesday the eleventh. This would let the doctors find out what damage, if any, had already been done to my brain.

Again, I asked the doctors if I could do a short jog that evening. And again, the answer surprised me.

"Sure, just take it easy. Don't do any hard workouts," they told me.

* * *

And so, while doing my streak-extending run of one mile on the treadmill, late on the evening of July 10, with Deb in bed because of her early shift the next day, I experienced a full-blown transient ischemic attack. At precisely 0.82 miles, my hearing went loud and screechy.

What's wrong with the sound on the television, I asked myself.

Even as the question was forming in my mind, I lost the coordination of my vision. I couldn't focus on the screen. What I saw wasn't double vision. Scrambled vision would be a more accurate description. The images in each of my eyes were convulsing wildly. It was as if someone had begun fiddling with the control knobs in my brain.

I lost my balance. Sliding backwards with my senses in disarray, I somehow managed to get off the treadmill before falling off. I slumped to the floor behind the machine. I crawled over to the couch and sat in stunned disbelief. There was a heavy tingling feeling in my left arm and shoulder. The treadmill was still humming as it slowly turned. The television was on, but I was not paying the slightest bit of attention to the program. All I knew was that I could see it and hear it normally.

After several minutes, when I felt sure that *it* was over, I got up and tried to walk. My legs were uncoordinated and clumsy. It was the same feeling I'd had on the morning we went to the ER. It seemed like quite a while had passed since the TIA had started, but it was probably not more than five minutes. Any lingering doubt I may have had that something was wrong with me was gone.

I carefully made my way down to my basement office, where I kept a blood pressure machine. With some difficulty, I got the cuff on my right arm. I checked my BP, as if I knew what I was looking for. I even recorded the result in a logbook I kept next to the machine. Then, in an epic sign of stubbornness—or maybe it was the stroke affecting my judgment—I decided it would be a good idea to go back upstairs and get on the treadmill, just to finish my mile and keep my running streak intact. All I could manage was a laboured walk at 2.5 miles per hour. I did 0.3 miles, to be sure that I had exceeded my one mile minimum for the day.

It did cross my mind at the time that perhaps my streak was already over, since my run for the day was not continuous. To be truthful, it wasn't even a run. I figured I could take these questions up later, on a point of principle, with the United States Running Streak Association, or USRSA, the governing body for running streaks. It never struck me as odd that there is such a thing as the USRSA.

Despite all the evidence to suggest a call to 911, I did nothing of the sort. Instead, I went to bed after deciding I would be fine. After all, I was scheduled to have an MRI at Foothills the next day. I did not wake Deb, who had already been sleeping for a few hours. However, at exactly 1:11 A.M., when she got up to go to the bathroom, I uncharacteristically woke up in a start. In the two minutes that she was out of the bedroom, I came to an important decision, a decision that may have saved my life. I knew that in a couple of hours she would get up and go to work, meaning that I might not get another chance to tell her what had happened.

"Deb, I have to tell you something. I've had a TIA. A minor stroke," I said.

I told her about how I'd lost control of my hearing and my vision, how I lost my balance on the treadmill, how I'd had that strange feeling in my arm and my leg. After discussing it for a few minutes, we decided that she would drive me to Foothills. We did not have to wait long in the ER, since they already knew my recent history. The on-call neurology resident, a polite young doctor named Andrea, led me to an examination room. As I followed her, I walked clumsily into the doorway. I think that said it all. She informed me that I was to be admitted to the stroke unit.

That was early in the morning of July 11. It was the beginning of what would be an extended stay in the Foothills Medical Centre. I was to be moved to Unit 100, on the tenth floor, as soon as a bed became available. In the meantime, I spent a long time waiting in a ward attached to the emergency room. Who knew they had so many beds back there?

Through the curtains, I listened to the activity all around me. I overheard a middle-aged man in the next bed who was having severe abdominal pain after a recent cancer treatment. With my faculties seemingly intact, I counted myself as pretty lucky.

I was taken for another CT scan. Then a resident from the stroke clinic came by and explained that I would be put on a statin drug and sent upstairs to the stroke unit shortly.

"But why are you sending me there?" I decided to ask, pushing back against my apparent fate. "I haven't had a stroke." I was still thinking that having a TIA meant I had somehow avoided having a stroke.

"Hmmm, what makes you think that?" she asked.

After another long wait, I had a visit from a doctor I would get to know quite well in the coming weeks and months. His name was Dr. Andrew Demchuk. He was accompanied by an entourage of residents and other doctors. Among their ranks, I recognized the young doctors I had already met. The first words Dr. Demchuk said did not endear him to me.

"Well, you may be fifty-six, but you have the arteries of an eighty-year-old."

"What do you mean?" I asked, in a curt tone. The stress of this ordeal was getting to me.

He explained his comment with reference to my age and my apparently good health. He had heard that I was a runner, and we talked about that. I explained that I had competed in road races as recently as three weeks ago, without incident, as if that would change his mind about my situation.

I was still grappling with the idea of taking drugs like statins to treat something I barely understood and, I assumed, did not apply to me anyway. I asked him about that.

"Oh, there's no question about it. You will be on a statin for the rest of your life," he said. He seemed surprised that I was even asking.

Late in the afternoon, I was moved up to the tenth floor, as promised. I spent a restless night in my new digs. It was odd that one of the first thoughts I struggled with that night was whether I could continue my streak. Since that would have meant jogging up and down the hallway next to the stroke unit, I had to accept that my streak was officially over. The irony that my modest streak and the invincible Ron Hill's streak had both come to an end in 2017 did not escape me. I wondered if there might at least be an annual prize for the most noteworthy end to a running streak.

The next day, I was sent for an MRI, as a complement to the CT scans that had already been done. The CT scans gave an overall picture of the arteries in my head and neck, allowing the doctors to identify the location and size of the blockage. The MRI would provide a picture of my brain, to show whether and how much damage the TIA (or TIAS) had caused in my brain.

As an engineer, I had been trained to rely on evidence. And yet, despite being presented with irrefutable evidence, such as pictures of my damaged brain, I spent my first day in the stroke unit in denial. I was still fuming about having been admitted at all. It wasn't in my plans.

What am I doing here? I asked myself, over and over. After all, I could function as normal. I could walk, quickly, up and down the tenth-floor hallways. Again and again, I paced the corridor to a window that overlooked the city to the north and east. I compiled a mental inventory of all the equipment that had been parked in that corridor, and all the posters on the wall, like an impromptu test of my mental faculties. I walked farther, exploring the other units on the tenth floor. I counted my steps, so I would know, more or less, how far I had walked. I ruled out the prospect of jogging, but for a time I considered it.

* * *

While I waited, another standard test had been ordered for me, an echocardiogram, or ECG. One of the first things the doctors wanted to do was rule out my heart as the cause of the blood clots being sent my brain. They sent me for this test soon after my admission to the unit. I was still feeling put out to be in the hospital, and yes, I was feeling quite sorry for myself.

Instead, this turned out to be a most curious and poignant episode. It was the first time, but not the last, that I felt an emotional connection with the caring people who populate this small city within a city that is the Foothills Medical Centre. I was wheeled to the ECG by a compassionate older man named Bill. He could see that I was scared about what was happening to me. Bill told me that he had suffered a major stroke seven years earlier, and then had a heart attack. We talked about his experience, and I shared my concerns about my TIAS and the drugs that I had started taking.

"Don't let this define you," Bill told me. I vowed that I would not, and I started to feel better about everything.

The technicians who ran the ECG further brightened my mood. The senior technician was a gentle, middle-aged man named Nasir. He was a quiet perfectionist. In fact, he reminded me of myself. Nasir was training a bright young doctor named Sarah, who was obviously keen to do her best on her rotation through this lab. Sarah had been charged with running my test. Nasir directed her with a firm but caring manner. I felt like an actor in a strange movie scene. He gave us each our instructions, all to make sure they could capture the best shots of my heart's inner chambers.

"Steve, move a bit to your left. Now Sarah, angle down a little—a little more—there, there. Perfect. Perfect! Steve, hold your breath—hold—hold—! Take the picture, Sarah! Yes! Steve, you may now exhale!"

Since Sarah's success depended on my performance, I did my best to play my part—holding my breath or exhaling or moving just as I had been instructed. I heard later that the ECG showed no anomalies. My first thought was to be happy that Sarah had done so well, due in part to my supporting role. Then I remembered to feel relief that we could rule out one potential source of my strokes.

A Brief Anatomy Lesson

TWO MAIN SETS OF ARTERIES feed blood to the human brain. At the front of the brain are the left and right common carotid arteries. The common carotids divide into the external and internal carotids. The external carotids supply blood to the face and scalp, and the internal carotids do the same for the front of the brain. The carotid arteries are big, as far as arteries go, at about six millimetres in diameter for the average adult male. More to the point, they account for about eighty percent of the total blood supply to our brains.

This story is more concerned with how blood is supplied to the back of our brains. Here, we find the left and right vertebral arteries—the verts. These major arteries run from a point behind the collarbones, up and through the vertebrae in our neck and into the back of the brain. The verts originate from a junction with the subclavian arteries, another pair of large arteries that deliver blood into the arms. The verts are smaller than the subclavians, at about three millimetres in most adults.

Because of my background as a chemical engineer, I am familiar with liquid flow in pipes. Right away, I noticed something intriguing about the junction where the verts originate. At that point, the verts branch vertically straight up from the horizontal subclavian. Generally, blood flow in arteries is smooth and orderly. The word for this type of fluid flow is *laminar.* In some situations, like when there is an arterial blockage, blood flow can become chaotic, or *turbulent.* When it comes to blood circulation, turbulent flow usually isn't desirable. I wondered whether the abrupt change in flow direction at the vertebral artery junction with the subclavian might also contribute to turbulent flow conditions. I will come back later to the reason this might be important in my case.

One fascinating aspect to the design of the arterial system feeding the brain is the amount of redundancy that is built into it. In most people, the left and right vertebrals do the same job. The two separate arteries meet up in the back of the skull to form the larger basilar artery. It is the basilar artery that supplies the remainder of the blood to the brain, about twenty percent of the total. There *may* be several other arteries that branch off from the verts, including the posterior inferior cerebellar artery, or PICA. May is the right word here, because while feeding the basilar artery is the main function of the vertebral arteries, everyone's specific vascular connections are different. The PICA is the largest artery that branches off from the vertebrals, and one of three main arteries that supply blood to the cerebellum.

The verts take a rather tortuous path to get from the subclavian artery to the basilar artery. There are holes in the column of vertebrae in the neck (the cervical vertebrae), called foramen. The vertebral arteries wind their way north through the foramen. Tucked in between the last vertebra and the basilar artery connection is the point where the branch to the PICA is normally found.

The vertebral/basilar artery network supplies blood to the back part of the cerebrum (the largest part of the brain), and to parts of the cerebellum (the smaller part of the brain, below and behind the cerebrum), as well as to the brainstem (a stalk-like structure that connects the brain to the spinal cord). The bodily functions controlled by the cerebellum are balance, coordination, and vision control, so it makes sense that as my left vertebral artery was gradually getting blocked, I had problems with those functions.

The concept of redundancy extends further than just between the left and right vertebrals. It also includes connectivity between the two sets of arteries feeding the brain; that is, between the carotids and the vertebrals. At the base of the brain, where the various arteries come together, there is a circle of connections between the carotid and vertebral arteries. This arrangement of communicating arteries is called the Circle of Willis, named for Thomas Willis, an English doctor who discovered it in the seventeenth century. Several other arteries meet up in the Circle of Willis and then take blood away to other parts of the brain. The reason for the Circle of Willis is quite simple and elegant. If any of the main arteries is blocked, or occluded, then the arteries that depend on the blocked artery can be supplied from somewhere else. In other words, blood can flow around the circle to get to its destination by another route.

* * *

This sounds like a lot of detail, and it is. It is challenging enough to explain arterial circulation of the brain from a lay person's perspective. But there is more, because most of what I have described applies to the average human brain. One of the genuinely surprising things I have learned during this adventure is that each brain has a unique configuration of arterial connections. My description of the typical connections does not apply to everyone. It may not apply to you and it certainly does not apply to me. And therein lies the root of my problem.

It turns out that there are a couple of differences in how my own plumbing works. First, my right and left vertebral arteries do different functions. They are *not* redundant. They do not join up to form the basilar artery. My right vert is smaller than normal and is dedicated to feeding the PICA. It serves no other function—it ends there. My configuration is not that unusual. Many people have an arrangement other than a textbook Circle of Willis. When the doctors talk to me about this, they refer to it as an *incomplete* Circle of Willis. It doesn't seem that this situation, having an incomplete Circle of Willis, is necessarily a big issue *per se*. Besides, there is no option to fix it, given the complexities involved. An incomplete Circle of Willis is likely something that would only ever be discovered in an autopsy.

What this all means for me is that I cannot be without my left vertebral artery, because it is the only one feeding blood to the basilar artery at the back of my brain. That is also why having this artery fully blocked becomes a significant problem. Unfortunately for me, that is exactly what has happened.

As for the location of the blockage in my left vertebral artery, it occurs at the point where the artery branches off from the subclavian. The doctors call this the proximal end, the part nearest to its origin. If a person is to have a blockage in their vertebral artery, that is probably the best place for it, since the higher up on the artery that a blockage is, the more challenging it would be to access, if the doctors were to decide to do something about fixing the blockage.

We would soon learn one other important thing that is working in my favour. In fact, it is an essential thing, because it is keeping me alive. And although I may be stating it more definitively than the doctors ever would, I believe I have running to thank for it.

Apprenticeships

BY 1990, MY THIRTIETH YEAR, I was well into my second decade as a runner. My youthful passion for the sport had never waned. As a result, running had gone beyond a casual pursuit and had taken a permanent place in my life. I had already experienced so much in and through running that it was becoming impossible to imagine myself being without it.

It is worth thinking about why we do a certain thing, especially if it is the type of activity that we feel is part of what defines us. I'm not sure I could have found satisfactory words to describe my feelings about running as a young adult. With the benefit of hindsight, I feel better able to do so now.

Running had arrived unannounced into my life. In no time, it had become part of my identity. Yet, until I set out to write these words, I had rarely stopped to figure out why or how this had happened. As my thirty-year-old self, I had not given it a lot of thought. I knew that this activity was *good* for me, on several levels. Was it a simple question of mechanics? Of giving this system—my body—a chance to work properly through regular use? That was certainly true, but it fell well short of a complete explanation of how running had become part of my being.

I was still involved in the process of discovery that had started when I took up running as a teenager. Fifteen years later, the goal of the discovery process had shifted. As I moved on from the mechanics of running and racing, I found that it had become an exploration of myself and my potential as a human being. I was enjoying many rewards that came from being a dedicated runner.

And what were those rewards? First, and most obviously, I valued the fitness results that running gave me. I define fitness as a state of balance between body and spirit. Running could bring me to a place of harmony, both within myself, and between myself and my external environment. This was unique to running; at least I had never experienced it from any other activity. At those moments, which almost always occurred while running outdoors, it was possible to lose myself in the regular rhythm of the physical activity. It was no longer necessary to think about what I was doing. The movement itself became effortless, almost hypnotic, as if my mind had entrusted my body to carry on with its task. Pain and discomfort were forgotten.

Second, I was enjoying running for its own sake. It was inherently valuable on its own. I knew that many people took up running in search of benefits that they had heard it might offer them. To me, this is a faddish view, one that puts running into the same category as the latest diet craze. It had never occurred to me to think of running as something I should do to achieve another goal, such as losing weight or socializing with a new group of friends. I had asked nothing from running, yet it was paying rich dividends.

Was running a form of prayer, or meditation? Maybe. I was somewhat jaded after my years as a devout Catholic kid. An altar boy, in fact. In the church, I found that the focus tended to migrate towards the formalities, the rules, the rote prayers. And for what goal? Delayed gratification. It seemed we were being offered a trade-off of benefits in this life for benefits in the next.

I could understand how some came to see running as a religious experience, even though it didn't seem to describe what I was experiencing. To me, the value of running was intrinsic to the activity. Once I had allowed myself to get into the rhythm of a run, usually after a couple of miles, I found that I would reach a state in which my mind could free itself from my body. It was as if the physical turns and straights I followed on the road were matched by the turns and straights in my mind. I learned not to set off with pre-conceived ideas of what I should think about. If I did, the thoughts simply flowed as they would anyway, and not necessarily as I intended. My mind pursued its own agenda. Decisions I was weighing, problems I had yet to solve, situations I was struggling with—they were all in play when I ran.

The world was often much easier to deal with after a run because I could see things more clearly. The results were immediate. I suppose that while that description might come close to the definition of prayer, there was a distinction in my mind, arising from the dislocation of when I might expect to reap the rewards. So, even if running didn't quite meet the definition of a religious endeavour, it certainly *was* spiritual. It was as if running had become a close friend, someone who was always there for me, someone whose sense of purpose was grounded in my wellbeing. There was nothing about me that this friend did not seem to know.

My internal flame burned brightest when I ran. Running did not just free my mind to explore new ideas—it engaged me on all levels. It opened my heart to being more empathetic in my interactions with other people. It liberated my spirit, letting me see myself at my most fundamental, maybe even at my most vulnerable or child-like. It isn't going too far to say that I could see myself in those moments, at my absolute finest. What a great thing it was to be able to bring some of those qualities back into my daily life.

Although I couldn't have put these ideas into words at the time, running was helping to transform me, over many years and miles, into the person I could be. I see now that the answers to the elusive questions—the important questions—of who we are, and what the meaning of our lives really is, are revealed to us only in brief moments. There is no timeline or roadmap for how we should progress towards our ultimate potential. One day, we find ourselves grown up and out of the innocent days of our youth. We are saddled with all sorts of expectations—in my case, as an employee, a husband, a father. To find a compass, a guide, or better yet, a portal that opens a path back to what is profoundly important in life would be quite remarkable. Actually, it would be invaluable. For me, running had become that portal.

* * *

It may seem incongruous to say that as my perceptions of the intrinsic value of running became clearer, I also came to appreciate the more tangible rewards that it offered. After all, I was a competitive runner, and for the competitive runner there is something elemental, something pure, about racing. Measuring yourself against the clock and against other competitors is the ultimate test. Even so, it took me some time after I started in the sport to find my place within its competitive borders. After my abbreviated turn in university athletics, I knew my days of track racing were over. Through my teens and early twenties, I had run in numerous road races, even several marathons, but it was not until my years in Edmonton that I began to capitalize on my base of fitness, and my growing confidence, to make road racing my primary interest.

Racing became the ideal platform for testing and improving

myself. Races were also a key part of the social circle for me and my Roadrunner teammates, and given the growing popularity of running, there was an ever-expanding calendar of events. I ran different race distances, honing my physical skills and sharpening my competitive instincts. I tried different race tactics: go out fast and ease off to a steady pace, hold myself back in the early going before adding pace, or aim for an even pace. What I was grappling with turned out to be an infinitely complex problem. How should I portion out my reserves of energy, so as to maximize my efficiency over the course, adapt to changing circumstances on the fly, and finish strong? Each outing was like a game of chess. Some factors were within my control, so I worked to improve my form. My talented teammates were a great resource and a constant source of inspiration and knowledge. I sought their advice, studied their tactics, and tried to put them into practice for myself. And I shared willingly of my own experiences.

As my performances steadily improved, I turned my mind to meaningful race goals. I chose my target races carefully and avoided the temptation of an endless cycle of training and racing. I had seen talented runners burn out through overtraining and too much racing. Some succumbed to injury and others gave up the sport altogether. There wasn't much risk of me falling into that trap. I was not a prodigy, and I didn't face that kind of pressure. I was the purest of amateurs, and I was already devoted to running for my own reasons. Besides, work schedules and obligations at home often intervened to prevent me from committing myself to too many races. Still, when I prioritized my efforts, in the good years I could compete in all the races I could handle. Even in the down years I made sure to enter a few races, because I knew that there was no better way to stoke my competitive spirit.

No matter how much I raced, for me it was less about the racing than about the training. I needed the discipline, and I welcomed the kinship. I was invested in the whole process, a process that usually had very little to do with a finisher's medal as its goal. Once I had dedicated myself to a training program, the result was important, but whatever happened on race day the effort was never wasted. I inevitably found satisfaction in the races I had done during my buildup, and I always had the companionship of my training partners as a consolation.

In subsequent years, I have stayed true to myself and followed my own path in the sport. I've been secure in the knowledge that the significant achievements in my life—and by that I don't just mean running achievements—subtly and surely were changing me, to the point that I became less focused on the result, and more on the positives that came from preparing myself to face such challenges in the first place. The satisfaction of achievements earned this way, with diligence and humility, last a lifetime. And even as a young man, I already counted myself as extremely fortunate in the tally of my achievements.

The balance between the spiritual and tangible aspects of running had come to symbolize the quest to realize my full potential, and to help answer the question of what gave my life meaning. I am not a philosopher, so I do not feel especially well-equipped to answer this question. But here, hindsight is valuable: it has allowed me to look critically at my personal values. Perhaps the lesson I've learned is that we should be mindful to make such assessments before unforeseen events rob us of the opportunity. As a thirty-year-old, just rounding into form as a competitive runner, as a professional engineer in possession of all his faculties, as a husband and new father, I certainly hadn't thought much about how I would face the prospect of losing something that I had come to take for granted. I doubt I was unique in this regard. If I had, I'm not sure I would have had an answer for vague hypotheticals. What I had come to know was that running was offering me its special rewards, its rich intrinsic benefits, without regard to speed or to the achievement of concrete goals. For the time being, I was content to keep riding that wave.

* * *

One tangible goal occupied me constantly through the 1980s and 1990s. I dreamt about running the Boston Marathon. It seemed that the idea had been there since I started running. I was aware of the legends and the history of this race, the oldest and most famous marathon of them all. Still, for much of this time I felt like I was doing my apprenticeship. I did not consider myself ready to attempt Boston. If someone had asked me if I was ready to run Boston, I might have given the same answer had they asked me if I was ready to make an assault on the peak of Mount Everest. Instead, Boston was a race I read about and studied. I did my homework by reading whatever I could about the race. Usually that was limited to back page coverage in the traditional sports pages. The race, and indeed the whole concept of marathon running, was still largely treated as a novelty.

To satisfy my curiosity, I subscribed to *Runner's World* magazine and searched for books that could fill in some of the gaps about this historic race. My well-used copy of Jim Fixx's classic book, *The Complete Book of Running*, now falls open to the pages where he describes—with the help of cute cartoon figures running across several pages—every mile and quirky feature of the marathon. For years, inaccurate distance markers and missing water stations were accepted as part of the defining character of the race. I read and re-read those descriptions, to the point that I knew the names of the shops in all the towns the race passed through. As if that would help. I memorized the geography and the topography, mile by mile. This obsession was like the one I'd had with the rules of hockey when I was nine years old.

I thought about the tactics that I would use, assuming I would someday run the race. For that, I bought a couple of other books that provided me with rudimentary training programs. These were just about the only sources of information that I could find. I knew runners that had run marathons, but I was not lucky enough to find someone who could give me tips on Boston. I had to figure it out myself.

The history of the Boston Marathon is intertwined with that other famous race, Hamilton's own Around the Bay Race. Both races were first contested in the 1890s. Many icons of distance running, including some legendary Canadians, had competed in both events. The lists of past winners in Boston and Hamilton include many names that I recognized, even idolized. There was Jerome Drayton, the top Canadian marathoner, the national marathon record holder, and the 1977 Boston winner. He was also a two-time winner of the Bay Race, in 1973 and 1974.

Even after my dream of running Boston moved into the realm of the possible, I felt far from ready. My experience of running a few marathons had left me with more questions than answers. So, I found other events to run—local 5k and 10k road races, and even some half marathons. Those were less popular at the time, though. I was content with a promise to myself that I would try Boston at some point in the future. In the meantime, I sharpened my skills.

For many years, there was another, more fundamental issue—my qualifying time. The Boston Athletic Association, the BAA, is the organization that manages the Boston Marathon. They have tinkered quite a bit with qualifying times over the years. They still do. One figure loomed large when I first entertained the idea of running the race: 2 hours and 50 minutes. Between 1980 and 1986, this was the qualifying standard for the race's open division. It had been tightened through the 1970s from 4:00 to 3:30, and then to 3:00, following the huge increase in the number of applications, which was due to growing interest in the race. While it was not out of the question that I could run a three-hour marathon, my results so far seemed to confirm that I had much learning to do. My apprenticeship was apparently not over.

By 1990, though, a window of opportunity opened. The BAA reversed course and eased its qualifying standard to 3:10, because as the race grew in stature, it attracted bigger sponsors. Bigger sponsors meant that the marathon could be better organized to handle the annual influx of runners, which had pushed the field size to almost ten thousand. While my personal best had dipped just under 3:00, I felt that further improvement would be needed before I was ready to accept the challenge. Still, the prospect of running the race had become more a question of when, rather than if.

* * *

The late 1980s and early 1990s were productive years for me at Shell. After more than five years, I had become bored with my work as a process control specialist. By then, I knew the managers in other technical departments well enough to drop hints that I was ready for a change. Soon enough, change came. I was offered the role of operations engineer, which put me right in the middle of the action in the refinery. This was a satisfying move and, even better, one that opened doors to other career paths. I collaborated daily with process economists, who dealt with complex questions of how to increase profitability of the plant, and I knew that was the right direction for me.

As it happened, I had worked closely on a few similar projects with one of the senior managers from Shell's Calgary head office. He had become a valued mentor and a friend. Demonstrating his confidence in me, he arranged for another shift in my career path. In 1991, with his encouragement and support, I was offered a move to Calgary, the city that was to become home to my family for many years. There, I would take on the job of preparing short-term operating plans for the company's western Canadian refineries, terminals, and pipelines.

As for the details of the move, I would be in the advance party. Shell wanted me to move a few months before Deb and Matthew. This made sense, as I could spend the time needed to start climbing the steep learning curve that came with the job. There was one other detail to consider. Deb was pregnant with our second child and was due to give birth that summer. We would be moving at almost the same time as her due date. She would also bear the burden of getting the house ready to sell and overseeing the packing in Edmonton. She had continued working at the Cross Cancer Institute through the spring, adding another dimension to an already complex situation. I made the trip back and forth several times, but it was Deb who pulled all the many details together and made it happen. I still have no idea how she managed to do it.

We bought a house in an older, established neighbourhood just south of downtown. As usual, Deb had done her homework in narrowing our search and finding us a suitable house. She did so just in time. We took possession of the house in July and our second son, Daniel, was born a few days later, in early August.

As 1991 ended, we were getting settled in a new city. Everyone was content at home. Deb and I looked to the future with optimism. I was busy at work, familiarizing myself with a corporate head office and getting to know the many contributors to the operating plans that I prepared every month. My job was everything I had been looking for. It was rewarding and challenging. It required strict attention to deadlines so that plans could be prepared and approved on schedule. Apparently, I would need all my technical skills and personal attributes to succeed in this role.

A Year to Remember

I HAD AN EARLY INTRODUCTION to the vibrant Calgary running community when I joined a Shell team for the 1991 Jasper–Banff Relay. Because the race happened around the same time as our move, it made what was already a hectic time a little more challenging. The race itself was memorable. We had a formidable team and finished second in the corporate division. I made the long drive to and from the mountain parks with Rob, a technologist from Shell's head office. We hit it off immediately. We became fast friends and frequent running partners from then on. Rob was an extraordinary runner, fast and efficient, with a superb marathon PB of under 2:30. As I mentioned earlier, he had one of the longest running streaks of anyone I knew.

I approached 1992 with a renewed passion for running. A frequent meeting place for downtown runners was the Eau Claire Y, a few steps from the beautiful Bow River. The Y was a couple of blocks from my office, which made it the logical choice as my running headquarters. It seemed there was always someone to connect with for an informal run at lunchtime or after work. I would often meet Rob or one of the other guys who had become friends since our move to Calgary. Doug was a strong runner with a great racing resume. He had a type-A personality when it came to running—he had to be in the lead. Tom was a triathlete. He was more relaxed about training paces, although he was more stressed about other things in life. My runs with Tom were often extended just to accommodate our engaging conversations.

Then there were the many colourful characters that I got to know through my visits to the Y. Fellows like Roy, a soft-spoken older gentleman, a runner, and a lawyer originally from Nova Scotia. He had been practising law in Calgary for years. I began to look for an open locker near his favourite—304—so we would have regular opportunities to chat. Roy would most often jog by himself along the river pathways at lunchtime, his competitive running days behind him. He would tell me, "The older I get, the faster I was." I feel like I now know what he meant.

Then there was Dwayne, a small-town Alberta farmer who worked in oilfield services. Dwayne's exploits were hilarious, bordering on the unbelievable. Once, he was hit by a car as he crossed Fifth Avenue, but he lived to tell the tale. Somehow, he ended up under the car, and he showed us the tire tracks across his chest to prove it.

"You should have seen the driver's face!" he said to the shocked crowd that had assembled near his locker to hear the story.

Among my new circle of running friends, Rob was the guy I enjoyed running with the most. He could handle any pace that was comfortable for me. I felt myself rising to this implied challenge as my fitness increased. Rob, Doug and I would often do a workout together. I knew I was in for an arduous run, and an extended lunch break, whenever we connected. Our preference was to run west along the Bow River, from the Y towards Edworthy Park. The path was in constant, heavy use by runners and cyclists. We were all attracted by the same thing—having the wide river by our side as it flowed east through the core of the city.

The distance to Edworthy was about seven kilometres, and we could count on getting there in less than thirty minutes. If we continued west, to the next convenient turnaround point at the Shouldice Pool, it would add a couple of kilometres to our outbound run. Or we could head up the gruelling, kilometre-long hill from the park to the neighbourhood of Wildwood. A full circuit of the hill takes nine or ten minutes if you are in good shape. We were. Many times, we would do a few hill repeats before heading back downtown. Inevitably, our pace on the return would increase, little by little, to something approaching an all-out sprint. I could count on Doug and Rob battling each other for the lead. I was usually content to let them beat each other up, while I did my best to hang on. I figured, no matter where I was in relation to them, I was getting huge benefits from the experience.

The results of my more intense training started to materialize right away. The first major event on the race calendar was the popular Police Half Marathon, held in late April. Half marathons—21.1 kilometres or 13.1 miles—were only starting to gain wide acceptance as a race distance. Before this one, I can't recall running a half since my days in Sarnia. In 1992, I was looking forward to the Police Half as a test of my fitness. As I had done often in the past, I let myself get caught up in the enthusiasm of a brisk early pace. The difference was, on this day I did not feel myself straining at all. I went with my gut and decided to maintain what would have normally been a suicidal pace in a half marathon. I got to the 10k mark on Memorial Drive in less than thirty-six minutes, bursting with energy. My watch was warning me that I had already crossed over into dangerous territory, but I began to feel that this might be a special day. Stop looking at it, I told myself.

The second half of the race included a steep hill on MacKay

Road at the 15k mark. I knew that my recovery would be shortened if I kept my effort steady, rather than my pace. That worked. I felt my strength return in a wave and I gathered myself for the last few kilometres. The field was getting quite strung out by this point, so I concentrated on the figure of the runner half a block ahead of me. This was made easier by long, straight stretches along Bowness Road. Now I had one tactic to the finish—push the pace as much as I could for as long as I could.

Don't you dare turn around, I muttered.

I rounded the last corner and saw the large clock above the finish line. Ignoring the numbers, I sprinted. It didn't register until I was walking through the chute that I had crossed the line before the clock reached 1:17. I finished in sixth place overall. Even as I heard my name called for a prize at the award ceremony, the reality had not fully sunk in. I was still feeling the thrill of the moment, high on a rush of adrenaline that had not yet subsided.

Later, as I relaxed on a lawn chair at home, sipping a beer in the warm spring sunshine, I replayed every minute of the race in my head. I began to comprehend what I had done. My daring start had led to a huge improvement in my previous best. I wondered if this might be the beginning of something special. I was filled with optimism, and I couldn't wait to race again.

Many local runners would be involved in the Jasper–Banff Relay in early June, but it didn't make sense for me to try finding a spot on a team. Committing to that race would mean a bigger issue on the home front, as it would consume the whole weekend and then some. Instead, I decided to run a smaller race in town, the Wood's Home 10k. I will not say that I was seeking to improve my chances in the race, but it didn't hurt that many of the top runners would be out of town. As it turned out, I won the race outright, in a new PB of 34:20. I started strong and led from start to finish. It was the first race I had ever won. I suppose in my records, there should be an asterisk next to that entry, given the extenuating circumstances, but a win is a win.

At that time, Rob was getting into ultrarunning. Over the next decade, he would become very accomplished at races longer than the marathon. In those early days, he would try to convince me to join him on his weekend training runs. That would have meant a four- or five-hour outing. I could never get my head around the commitment needed to run for that long. Besides, I would have had to convince Deb that this was how I should be spending my weekends. We had lists of better things to do. As a compromise, Rob and I came up with an arrangement where we would run together for two or three hours at a time. He tapped other friends to take similar shifts, so in the end, everyone was happy. For me, those miles were a solid foundation, because the more running I did with Rob, the better.

The K–100 Relay in late June was next on my race calendar. I ran for a second time on the Shell corporate team. We finished third in our division, and fourteenth overall in a field of nearly two hundred teams, a great accomplishment given the depth of some Calgary corporate teams. I ran the intimidating ninth stage, which at 19.5 kilometres was the longest one in the race. It also had a daunting hill towards the end. I finished seventh, a shockingly good result for me. I was ecstatic.

To add some interest, on that day Rob ran the individual ultra, a fifty-mile race that had been added to the relay. Because it started at the end of Stage 4 and followed the relay route, I was able to see him through the day. While Rob was struggling mightily towards the end of the race, he won it handily. My friend's gritty performance was awe-inspiring.

The focal point of my summer racing season was the Calgary Marathon, which coincided with the start of the annual Calgary Stampede in early July. My K–100 result suggested that I was fit for the marathon. I had a couple of weeks to recover before the race. The route was flat and fast and was becoming quite familiar to me after a year in the city. The possibility of hot, humid conditions was a concern. Still, everything seemed to be coming together at the right time, and my race performances so far for the season were encouraging. I began to taper my mileage and made my last preparations for the race. For his part, Rob decided to tackle the marathon at the last minute. It was a courageous move. Our mutual friend Doug would also be running, as would some other friends and work colleagues.

I went through my final planning for race day. Then everything just about fell apart.

Our son Daniel, who was by then nearly a year old, had been a sound sleeper most of the time. However, on this night, he had some unknown issue that kept him up until the early hours. I was reduced to lying in bed with my eyes open, thinking about what this would do to my marathon in a few hours. I never expected to get a good sleep the night before a big race, but this was a whole new problem. I made no secret of my frustration to Deb, but there was nothing to be done.

Finally, Daniel quieted down, and I fell asleep. Too soundly, as it turned out. In addition to my other troubles, I had set my alarm incorrectly and it did not wake me up when I had planned. The only thing that saved me was my decision to take a cab to the race. The sound of the driver honking his horn was my alarm. At first, the sound was part of a dream, but as the cobwebs slowly cleared it dawned on me what had happened. I leapt out of bed, totally skipped my normal race day breakfast, and jumped into the car for the short ride downtown. Still half asleep, I stowed my bag at the Y, where the marathon would start in a matter of minutes. I headed to the start line, believing that my day was ruined.

I need not have worried. Missing my routine and my breakfast appeared to do me no harm. Instead, the early miles of the race were quite pleasant. The conditions were ideal, with mild temperatures, light cloud cover, and no wind to speak of. A bit of banter with the runners around me helped settle me down, and I began to forget about my chaotic start. I got to the 10k mark in 39 minutes. The pace felt effortless. Be patient, I reminded myself. I reached the half in 1:23, feeling relaxed and comfortable. I knew I was well placed in the field and holding my own against other racers, several of whom I recognized. Rob and Doug were up the road, and I wondered how they were doing. I would have to wait until the 25k turnaround point on Bowness Road to find out. When I saw them heading back towards the finish, they were both looking strong and well-positioned in the top ten. I counted another ten runners or so before I too made the turn for home.

I made it to the twenty-mile mark in 2:07, and the 40k mark in 2:40. I knew I was losing time on the final stretch on Memorial Drive, but I tried to remind myself that this was just another long run and that I had a home field advantage.

"Just one more run back to the Y," I whispered over and over, like my mantra for the race. I gave myself permission to take a couple of walk breaks through the water stations. I crossed over the pedestrian bridge at Tenth Street, knowing it would only be a couple more minutes to the finish. My last mile was going to be slow. I tried to forget about my pace and keep moving forward. I spotted the banner indicating the finish and I made a token sprint. I crossed the line in 2:51 and change. It was a personal best by more than seven minutes. I finished twentieth overall.

The first person I saw at the finish line was Rob. I did not know yet how he and Doug had done. He didn't hide his competitive nature.

"What the hell happened to you?" he asked, matter-of-factly.

I mumbled something about my race time being a huge PB, and

I started to explain the less-than-ideal start to my morning. That was all irrelevant, of course.

In his own, rather harsh way, Rob was right. Based on our recent training history, my performance should have been better—maybe much better. It was, after all, my most legitimate shot at the marathon result I always thought I should have had. As for my training partners, they both hit their targets. Doug finished fourth, and Rob was sixth, in a strong field. I marvelled at how he had managed to do that, two short weeks after a fifty-miler.

Depending on how one predicts race performances, I should have been capable of running a marathon in the 2:40–2:45 range. True, I did not deliver on my potential on that day in July 1992, leaving five or even ten minutes on the table. Maybe it was due to the chaos of the night before. Maybe it was a lack of some element in my preparation. Or maybe, as I was beginning to suspect, the marathon was just not my race. More than once during our many runs together, Rob said to me, "For someone who trains at the level you do, I don't understand why your race performances aren't better." Perhaps this was never truer than on that day. As a result, I filed the race away, under the category of disappointing performances. It was not Rob's comment at the finish line that did it. I secretly did feel that this was my big chance.

I should add, though, that as time has gone by, I look back on that race differently. I now consider it to be a good, but not great, performance. I ran a reasonably steady pace, and I did nothing dumb. No one should ever be unhappy with a seven-minute marathon PB. I had averaged 6:32 per mile for 26.2 miles that day. In modern units, that is 4:04 per kilometre for 42.2 kilometres. Probably not more than one percent of marathon runners can make that claim. Still, I am left to wonder how I might have done that morning had I been armed with some of the mental tactics that I would add to my toolkit years later. But on the day, and given the rough start that I had, I am satisfied that it was a fair indication of my potential.

So, 1992 was a year in which the stars aligned for me. I recorded strong performances in all the major road race distances. I set substantial personal bests in the 10k, the half marathon and the marathon. I had done very well in the mountain relay. It was a year to remember.

* * *

Not all the memories from 1992 are positive. My father continued to sink deeper into the clutches of alcoholism. It cost him his job at the post office, and after a protracted dispute over his sick pay, much of his dignity. He retired with a full pension and started spending his time and most of his money in local watering holes. His health deteriorated because he was eating less and less as he drank more.

My in-laws, Kurt and Lisa, lived in Toronto. Kurt had recently retired and was looking forward to pursuing a long list of interests and hobbies. Kurt would often write us letters in his neat, distinctive hand. We suspected something was wrong, when his letters showed that he was having trouble keeping his writing within the lines. We thought he might have suffered a minor stroke. The diagnosis, when it came in the spring, was much more serious. Brain cancer.

I loved Kurt dearly, maybe because he was in some ways the opposite of my own father. He was meticulous, organized, and practical to a fault. Like Dad, he loved music, but it was classical or jazz rather than pop. I suppose their musical tastes might have aligned somewhere around Frank Sinatra or Tony Bennett. Kurt drank, but always in moderation, and typically only in the form of a glass of sweet white German wine with dinner, or a tiny sip of fine cognac.

It was difficult to be so far from Toronto while Kurt was sick.

I saw him and Lisa a couple of times as they suffered through his horrible and rapid decline. Deb was an only child, and we were on the opposite side of a huge country with two young children of our own. The situation was especially hard on Deb's mother. We were shocked at how fast Kurt went downhill—it was heartbreaking. Deb did what she could for her parents during that terrible time.

We knew by midsummer that the end was near. I had signed up for the ten-mile Robert Hamilton race in late August. I guess I was hoping to add a PB at that distance to my earlier accomplishments, as a way to cap off an unforgetable year of racing. On race morning, I woke up to an unusually early snowstorm that left a couple of inches of snow on the ground. I persevered, leaving the house early to get to the race, even though I probably should have skipped it. My results were less than stellar, but maybe this was to be expected, considering the treacherous conditions.

As it turned out, the race was irrelevant. What I did not know was that as I was running and making the slow drive home, Deb had received the call from Toronto that she was dreading. Her father had slipped into a coma. She was advised to catch the next available flight. Because it was before the days of cell phones, she had no way to reach me while I was out of the house. She had frantically made her preparations to fly back to Toronto, and she left the house as soon as I got there. Kurt died while she was in the air.

Kurt's passing was a profound shock for Deb and me, even though we had known the end was coming. He had always been good to me, and he was a wonderful father to my wife. To this day, I have kept the blue T-shirt from the 1992 Robert Hamilton race. It sits on the bottom shelf in my closet, unworn, because it never felt right to either wear it or get rid of it. I suppose I keep it as a reminder to be thankful when things seem to be going well, because those stretches do not last forever. That shirt seems to have taken on more significance in the last couple of years.

Mission Accomplished

THINGS TEND TO GO IN CYCLES. And maybe it is hardest thing of all to stay at a peak already reached. Whatever the case, by 1993, my running seemed to have already moved off the highs of just a year earlier. I did manage a couple of decent races—I went under 1:20 once again in the Police Half Marathon, and I won the Wood's Home race for the second year in a row—but those were to be the highlights of the year.

My priorities had shifted. Deb and I had two young sons to attend to. My workload at Shell had continued to increase. The monthly operating plans I prepared were essential to the business, but the timelines were unforgiving. As a result, I was putting in a significant amount of overtime. There was no alternative. I met the challenge I had taken on.

To add to my list of distractions, I enrolled in a part-time Master of Business Administration program at the University of Calgary. If I were to see it through to its conclusion, which was by no means certain at the beginning, this would mean several years of concerted effort to complete the necessary course work. It would also require a willingness by my young family to make plenty of sacrifices. I am not sure what motivated me to take on this burden, although it had been in my mind for several years as an opportunity worth pursuing. I liked the academic environment, and I liked learning new things. Once again, my personality traits of curiosity and diligence seem to have conspired against me!

The next few years were a down time for running, due to my MBA studies and one other factor. During this period, I ran about four times a week on average, and I did very little racing. In 1995, I set my sights on one goal race for the season, the Calgary Stampede Run-off 10k. I figured I could improve my result by including weight training and core strength exercises as a supplement to the running I was doing. For help with this, I worked with the strength coach for the Calgary Flames. After three months on his regimen, I ran the race and finished in a disappointing time. At the time, I was upset with how badly I had faded in the second half. If I had considered the bigger picture and the juggling act I was doing, I should not have been surprised. I had been doing no speed work, and overall, my mileage was not where it needed to be. But it is not easy to see such extenuating factors while you are fully occupied.

The second and perhaps bigger factor came in 1996, when I changed jobs. For a year or two, I had been restless at Shell. The company was between big projects and was not giving me much evidence that it had my long-term interests in mind. I started looking around. Finally, after a frosty exchange with my boss, I phoned the manager at a small energy consulting company whom I had met a year earlier. I was not sure what I intended by phoning him. I suppose I was going to let him know that I would be interested in a job, should anything become available. To my surprise he suggested getting together to discuss it. We met the next morning for coffee.

In fairly short order, I joined the firm, Purvin & Gertz, as an associate. At the time, I really did not know much, if anything, about the consulting business, so it was a daunting prospect. However, my experience at Shell had set me up well for the kind of work that this firm specialized in. My move was to be the beginning of a long, rewarding and ultimately successful career as a consultant.

It also meant that for the time being, I was overloaded. I was in the middle of my MBA program and had taken on a job that required many hours of fastidious work each week. Besides that, I had another steep learning curve to climb. In a field that defines success by hours billed, and in which associates like me were the foundation for the detailed analytical work done by the firm—we called it the heavy lifting—I was, to put it mildly, thrown into the deep end.

I soon learned that the consulting business is not for everyone. Our company president used to joke that we were always one month away from going out of business. There seemed to be little chance of that, as the firm had an enviable global reputation. My new colleagues were capable and welcoming. I hit it off with them from the start. Even better, I appreciated the diversity that came with working with our clients on a broad range of projects. Perhaps I was naïve, but it never occurred to me to worry about where my next job was coming from.

With the added burden of learning a new job—actually a new career—my focus on competitive running took a further hit. However, in what was an astounding paradox, the important role that running occupied in my life was enhanced, rather than diminished, during this chaotic period. In fact, it was during this time that the true value of running for me was solidified. I found that whatever else I had on my plate, I had to set aside some time each week for myself, and running was the obvious place to take refuge.

I came to depend on a few familiar and treasured running routes. One of my favourites I called the Stampede Loop. Depending on which way around I ran it, I would either head east from my house to the Elbow River, or north to the Bow River. I would follow that river to its confluence with the other at Fort Calgary Park. Either way, the sights were marvelous, through the heart of downtown or past Lindsay Park and the Stampede Grounds. The fort was both the farthest point from home and the lowest point of elevation on my route, but for me it was the highlight. I find something calming about seeing the water from the two rivers come together at that spot. From there, it was all uphill to get back home, and if I had run in the counterclockwise direction, saving the Fourteenth Street hill for last, I knew the last couple of kilometres would be tough. But whichever direction I went, having the rivers at my side seemed to provide a perfect counterbalance to the heavy demands that my work and school were putting on me.

If I chose to run south from home, I would soon join up with the southbound part of the pathway system in River Park. From there, it was clear running all the way to Fish Creek Park if I felt up to it. More often than not, I would run past the Glenmore Athletic Park to North Glenmore Park, taking in the beautiful vistas across the Elbow River valley and the reservoir along the way. A loop of the reservoir made for a superb long run. At the far end of the circuit, reached by heading down to a footbridge and then across the marshy Weaselhead Flats, I could almost be convinced that I was no longer in the city. Quiet winter mornings were the best, with my footfalls making the only noise as they crunched through a fresh snowfall. The south side of the reservoir was picturesque. I ran through a birch forest and past the Glenmore Sailing Club, before heading north to reach Heritage Park and the pathway that would take me back home.

* * *

With some forward planning and a little luck, a path to the 2001 Boston Marathon presented itself. After a monumental effort, involving sacrifice by the whole family and classes four nights each week, I finished my MBA program in 1998. I started filling the extra time that this created by doing some targeted training, including decent long run mileage on the weekends. It was a major step to commit to a marathon, particularly since almost six years had passed since I'd achieved my PB. By targeting the 2001 race, I could move up to the masters division, and gain some additional relief in the entry standard, which had been adjusted once more by the BAA, to an almost pedestrian 3:20.

I began the tactical planning. Given the calendar for Boston entries, I would need to choose a marathon that was scheduled shortly after September 2000. My preference was for a race that was not likely to be affected by my nemesis—hot weather. I wanted a race that was Goldilocks-sized, neither too big nor too small. And ideally, it should not be too far from home. A race that checked all my boxes was the Victoria Marathon, which would take place on the Thanksgiving weekend in early October.

My training calendar for the months leading up to the Victoria race—one of the few periods where I did keep meticulous records—is full of tiny writing that describes the details of every run and training session. Knowing that I had fallen short on some element or other when training for previous marathons, I was determined to reach the start line in Victoria totally prepared. I signed up for interval training at Lindsay Park. These were the sessions where I met Mahedi and several other runners who would become great friends and frequent training partners. We were like-minded in our approach to training, born out of a shared passion for running. We all wanted to be better racers, and we knew what was required to reach that goal. The sessions were just what I needed, a complement to the mileage I was doing on the roads. Over that spring and summer, I steadily built my base. I did many long, solitary runs. I think I covered every inch of the river pathways. I made sure to include lots of quality workouts, and I ran several strong races, all with one intermediate goal in mind.

* * *

My brother Paul was a great runner. There was no doubt about that. His personal bests made mine look ordinary. I had no idea how many city championships and Ontario high school wins he managed to accumulate. His varsity athletics career at McMaster was as impressive as mine was forgettable. Although his specialty on the track was 800 metres, he could run just about anything. On the road, he excelled at the 5k distance, but he raced and won 10k races all over Southern Ontario during the 1980s and 1990s.

Fast forward to 2000. My juvenile jealousy about Paul's superior running ability had long since softened. That summer, I was deep into my Victoria Marathon buildup. I was doing a lot of mileage, tempo work and interval training. In August, we stopped in southern Ontario for a vacation trip that would include a few days in Bobcaygeon. We wanted the kids to enjoy an Ontario cottage experience, like we had when we were young. While we were there, we made obligatory visits to Hamilton and Toronto. It occurred to me that there might not be a better opportunity to challenge Paul to a head-to-head contest. Although he was still running and racing at a high level, this seemed like the narrowest gap that had ever existed between us.

I asked him to find a race where we could do battle. Plans were put in place for us to run in the Niagara-on-the-Lake Peach Festival race. He had run this race before, so he would have the home field advantage. Anticipation built in the days before the race. Paul's wife Shelley and their three daughters, and my sister Carolyn and her three sons, all got into the spirit of the showdown.

Race morning was warm and humid—typical summer weather

in Ontario. I had to concede another point to Paul. Still, I was confident about my chances. It was a frenzied scene in my parents' house as we organized the convoy of minivans. Adults and kids ran in and out the front door, and up and down the stairs, getting all the details organized. I had already given up on my usually deliberate race preparations. With no time to spare, we got people and gear loaded into the vehicles and set off.

We settled into the drive, with me behind the wheel and Deb beside me. It was the first chance we had to relax since we had woken up. A few minutes later, I had a sinking feeling.

"Oh, damn!" I said.

"What's wrong?" Deb asked.

"I think I forgot my running shoes."

"You've *got* to be kidding," she said, with a look that said she had seen this movie before.

"No, I'm sure I left them in the house." As I got my race kit together, I had reminded myself to make one more trip upstairs to get my shoes from my suitcase. In all the excitement I never did it.

I announced to the passengers behind us what had happened. Then I heard my mother's spontaneous laugh coming from the back seat.

"Oh Steve! You've never changed." She was overcome with laughter, thinking about the countless times I had left the house for school, only to come back seconds later to get whatever it was that I had forgotten that day.

When we got to the race, accusations flew from Camp Paul that I had been afraid to go through with this long-awaited and much-hyped showdown. We rummaged through his van to see if a spare pair of his shoes could be made to work. That was unlikely, since my feet are two sizes bigger than his. The showdown was not to be.

"We should at least use the race entry that we've already paid for," someone suggested.

"But who would be able to do it?"

I wonder if our twelve-year-old son Matt felt the multiple sets of eyes that turned towards him. Despite his initial reluctance, he agreed to run the 5k race with Deb. I was relegated to holding the bags and cheering from the sidelines. In the end, I'm quite sure that Paul would have won our battle. He ran an impressive time that I don't think I could have bettered. But I never admitted that to him.

As a small reward for Matt's good sportsmanship, he won a draw prize after the race. He left happy. He didn't want the race shirt, which was, naturally, peach-coloured and had cute peaches running across the front. It became my consolation prize. That, and the nagging thought that just maybe I really had wanted to forget my shoes so the race would not happen.

* * *

Our visit to Ontario allowed us to see for ourselves how much Dad had declined. Alcoholism had taken total control of his life. By then, he was eating almost nothing and was withdrawing into his own little world. He had been admitted to hospital once, where he spent a week in detox. Although he began to show some improvement, he took up his old habits as soon as he was released. It seemed that he was in a terminal decline.

The city, too, seemed to be suffering a sympathetic fate. Intense competition from offshore steel producers had undermined Hamilton's industrial foundation. Successive rounds of job cuts had done little to stem the losses at Stelco's main Hilton Works plant. Dofasco was faring better, but only just. To the outsider, as I then was, it was impossible not to notice an ever-widening gap in prosperity between Hamilton and Calgary. My adopted hometown was becoming a thriving, cosmopolitan place—one of the most livable cities in the world. By contrast, Main Street and King Street, the two vibrant

Hamilton arteries I remembered so well from my childhood, were turning into endless strips of urban decay. My old neighbourhood, now devoid of the friendly faces that I had grown up with, seemed somehow to be a less welcoming, much reduced version of itself.

In Toronto, the news was better. After my father-in-law's tragic illness and death, my mother-in-law, Lisa, had found a new partner. Andy was a gentle and generous man. He ran a precision machine shop in the city. We enjoyed our visits to their home. The boys and I were fascinated by his ingenuity with machine tools. And Deb and I were relieved that her mother was in a stable, long-term relationship. She was happy. She and Andy belonged together.

* * *

I stood on the start line in Victoria's beautiful Inner Harbour, in ideal race conditions. I was strangely calm. It was the calm that comes before a meeting with destiny. Barring a catastrophe, I would soon achieve my Boston Marathon qualifying standard of 3:20. I was confident I could go faster, and I had an incentive to do so: faster qualifiers would earn a more favourable starting position in April. To improve my chances, I seeded myself at the front of the three thousand runners assembled on the road. Today, I wanted every possible advantage.

The early miles slipped by easily. I felt detached, more like a spectator than a racer. My split time at 10k was under forty minutes. Too quick. It was the adrenaline, with an extra boost from the oxygen-rich atmosphere at sea level. I throttled back, knowing that it would be suicidal to try and hold this pace. The field was already spread out, meaning I could watch the road ahead of me for hazards, and attack the shortest line through the curves. I found my rhythm. I took water at each station, and for the first time in a marathon, I carried energy gels. I had been practicing with them in my training runs, but their gooey consistency occasionally made me gag. I hoped they would help me in the latter stages of the race.

I recall very little until the 35k mark. A time check there jolted me with the realization that I had a good chance to meet my optimistic target, a three-hour finish. Even with the gels, I had reached the point of exhaustion that inevitably came in a marathon. My pace was fading, and it became a case of trying to minimize the damage. All morning I had managed to hold off thoughts of what the future might hold, but in these final kilometres my brain struggled to stay engaged. In my mind's eye, I was already seeing images of myself in Boston. I urged my legs on, drawing whatever energy I could from the growing crowds as I approached the harbour.

Keep it together, I told myself. This is what all the training miles were for.

Finally, I saw the legislature building. I rounded the last corner before the finish straight and I sprinted on rubbery legs. It was an involuntary response more than a necessity. I finished in forty-fourth place, and a full hundred seconds before the clock reached three hours. These were satisfying numbers, but totally irrelevant. Far more important was how I had done against my qualifying standard. That I beat decisively, by almost twenty-two minutes.

I searched for Deb and the boys in the bustling finish area. I was exhausted but elated, knowing I had done everything possible to ensure myself of a good placing in Boston. I wanted to share this feeling, and to hear their stories, too. While I was on the road for my race she had taken on a couple of challenges of her own. This was a period when she had also applied herself to training and competing in triathlons. So, she took the opportunity of our time in Victoria to run in the 8k individual race. Then, she ran with the boys in the kids' race, doing the most important job of all—holding onto everyone's gear and clothes. It was quite a morning for all of us.

We flew home, everyone pleased with their results. I was

incredibly happy and bursting with confidence. My race wasn't perfect, but this was the result I had planned for, and the one I felt I needed to commit to Boston. Before I could even begin to think about changing my mind, I mailed in my race entry the next morning and set myself on the path to be on the start line in Hopkinton, Massachusetts in six months. I vowed to continue the same program elements that had got me this far, and I hoped that neither work nor injuries would get in the way.

My weekly track sessions at Lindsay Park became a core part of my training program and they were great fun besides. I gave these workouts my total effort, alongside my training partners. There was a certain code of honour about these sessions. Everyone shouldered their responsibility, taking their turn in the lead. We worked as a unit, supporting each other without words. Many times, I would jog from home to the session and back again when we were done, just to put more miles in the bank. Although my winter training schedule was onerous, mainly because I was doing most of my long runs alone, I took confidence from the fact that I was getting through it. Having access to the track as an option for long runs was a bonus, for the handful of days when the Calgary winter weather was simply unbearable.

As winter slowly turned to spring, I felt my strength building on the back of 90- to 110-kilometre weeks. For a short time, I shed other responsibilities, leaving only work and training. I dug deeper than I had ever done before. Learning from Victoria, I wanted to be stronger towards the end of the marathon, and for that, there was only one answer. It was all about the miles, about the time spent on my feet. I felt that I was in the best shape of my life, and I secretly hoped that I could hold it all together until mid-April.

Besides the mileage, my other numbers were encouraging. I signed up for a master's mile in late February, on the same track that we were using for our interval sessions. My coach, Ray, was full of advice, yelling last-minute tips even as I was taking my place on the starting line. Under his watchful eye, I ran 5:04 and finished third, a result we were both happy with. A couple of weeks later, I knocked out twelve 400-metre repeats—my all-time favourite workout—each in 73 to 75 seconds, chasing my training partner Vince. That night, I was invincible. My last data point before Boston was the annual St. Patrick's Day 10k race. I cruised to a fifth-place finish, and my time of 35:34 felt effortless. A colour picture in the next day's Calgary Sun shows me taking off from the front row of a sun-drenched start line, looking fit and confident. I was ready. It was time to turn a dream into reality.

* * *

It was disorienting to finally experience something that I had dreamt about for a quarter century. My mind was crammed with a thousand simultaneous thoughts: the traditions of Boston, the personalities, details of the route from Hopkinton to Copley Square, the perplexing course profile, contingencies for weather and other imagined risks. The Newton hills were what many Boston runners feared, but it was the overall net elevation drop—about 140 metres—and the early downhill miles that worried me more. Even so, reading about these issues and experiencing them first-hand would be quite different. If I had been pressed to declare a goal, I would have predicted a time close to what I had done in my qualifying race. Anything faster seemed unlikely, given the distinctive features of the Boston course.

It was a special trip. All four of us made the trip east and we stayed in a hotel a short walk south of the Boston Common. The race expo in the World Trade Center was huge. Intimidating. Navigating the halls full of gear and race history was a necessary part of the process. Still, I stressed over the thought of being on my feet too much. My typical pre-race nerves were working overtime. Deb wanted to see all of it and scolded me for being a grouch. I was relieved to get my bib safely in hand—number 2215, corral 2—so we could head back to the hotel. I felt better if I did a casual jog the day before a marathon, so Deb and I went out for a couple of miles around the Common. Anxious runners were everywhere. We had an early pasta dinner and retired to bed for what was to be a sleepless night.

On race day, Deb and the boys would wait for me at the finish line. I was up in the dark and did my best not to wake them. Boston is somewhat unusual, being a point-to-point marathon—the logistics of getting to Hopkinton meant an early start. It was cool at 8 A.M. as I nervously joined the well-organized queues for the buses that would drive us west from the Common.

It was impossible to know what awaited me. I made a bit of polite conversation with the runner next to me on the bus. He was a Boston veteran. While I was interested in his story, I was only half listening. I was past the point of absorbing any more information. The ride seemed to take forever, accentuating the obvious fact that we would run a long way to get back into the city today.

The athletes' village at the Hopkinton High School would be our temporary camp while we waited for the noon start time. Suddenly, as I stood in the place where so much running history had been made, the task before me felt very real. Next to the iconic "It all starts here" sign, I sensed the presence of the greats who had stood in this town square before me. On any other day, it would have been pleasant to wander through this quaint New England town. But on this cool April morning, other business had brought me here. The weight I had been carrying for so many years seemed to have gotten much heavier.

Most runners occupied themselves with staying warm. Given our long wait in the village, I forced myself to eat a bagel, a banana, and a little yogurt, even though I had no appetite. I went through a version of my pre-race routine, rationalizing that even if it were less than ideal it would have no impact on the outcome anyway.

I finished my preparations, wrapped myself up in a generous pile of spare clothes, and closed my eyes. I tried to relax, but my mind was already racing. At about 11 A.M., thirty minutes before the mass exodus to the start area on Main Street, there was an increase in the energy level around me, unlike anything I had ever felt before. The tension was palpable. The air crackled with the electricity generated by fifteen thousand penned runners. It was extraordinary. A noisy crescendo was reached, which could only be relieved by our slow, anxious walk to the starting corrals.

Despite the cool temperature, I opted for a singlet and shorts. I put on a cap, covered my ears with a headband, and chose a pair of thin wool gloves. I wore my favourite shoes, the Asics DS-Trainer. I counted on my winter training base and a modest warming that had been forecast though the morning. That would turn out to be a good call.

News helicopters buzzed overhead. I immersed myself in the nervous energy that had enveloped me. Runners were flush with adrenaline in these last few moments before the start. I tried to convince myself that this was just another race, but there was no denying it: I was about to start the most famous race in the world.

I heard the gun, but it was at least ten seconds before I had a vague feeling of moving forward. Hooting and hollering erupted. Unlike some of my fellow runners, I concerned myself more with not tripping than with celebrating. It took me nearly a minute to cross the start line, still in a slow shuffle. I did my best to resist the momentum of the thousands of runners behind me as I searched in vain for a bit of running room. Gaining speed, we began to negotiate the first few hundred metres, the most steeply downhill section of the whole course. I was not ready for the narrowness of the road. It was chaotic. Some runners freewheeled down the shoulder. Others took to the treed hills on either side of the road for bladder relief. My instincts as a high school cross-country athlete kicked in. I put my elbows out.

Lift your feet, I told myself. Don't brake on the hills. Conserve energy!

Looking ahead, I saw nothing but bobbing heads stretched to the horizon. The steepness of the hill and the tight confines of the road made me feel that I was a cork floating down the rapids of a raging river. By the time the river flowed into Ashland, the field was settling down. It was finally possible for me to do a check on my pace and form, having found some real estate to run in. I felt myself getting into a rhythm as I warmed up. I favoured the left side of the road, avoiding both the shoulder and the crown of the road. I did some early scouting of the water stations. One side of the road, then the other. Okay, no worries there.

I looked around at the rural stretch of Route 135 that would bring us through Framingham, then Natick, then Wellesley, in the first half of the race. I was struck by the juxtaposition of thousands of marathoners—all moving as fast as possible—and the bucolic scenery that seemed to be inviting us to slow down. I tried to recall the checkpoints that I previously knew by heart, but those names would not have made any difference even if I could pick them out. Instead, I took brief glances at the imposing nineteenth-century homes, the light industrial businesses, and most noticeably, the growing crowds. I wanted to have some visual memories from this experience.

At first, I was vaguely aware of the thousands who turned the marathon into an annual Patriots' Day party, in which we were the entertainment. Then I remembered that I was supposed to be enjoying this. It was no longer about surviving in the tumultuous river of runners. I noticed the little kids who held out orange slices and jellybeans for us. Although I declined their handouts, I gave a few of them the high fives they were hoping to receive from us, the runners. I passed the 10k banner in just over forty minutes. Fast, but probably okay, taking the frenetic downhill start and my high adrenaline into account. By then I was comfortable stashing my gloves in the waistband of my shorts and tossing my headband away.

We passed a tranquil lake as we entered Natick. Was it Cochituate? Conchitate? Something like that. My mind drifted as I pondered where that name might have come from.

I caught snippets of conversation from the spectators. An hour into the race, I overheard a man tell his friend, "These runners have absolutely no chance of winning." I only had time to shoot him a quizzical look as I ran past. He was right, of course, but he might have liked to know that by being there at all, I had already won. Besides, I was working every bit as hard as the speedsters up front. I might have also mentioned that having already passed the 15k mark, I was doing fine. Better than fine. His odd comment was just what I needed to strengthen my resolve.

I began to appreciate what a major international event this was. In what I considered a showy demonstration of patriotism, I had asked Deb to sew small Canadian flags onto my hat and my singlet. As the crowds grew larger and noisier, I could hear shout-outs to runners from many countries. Someone shouted towards me.

"Go Canada!"

I gave a modest wave in response. Only then did I notice the runner to my left, decked out from head to toe in red maple leaves. I guessed that the cheer was probably not for me after all, but I helped myself to some of the ambient energy. (I later counted fifty-four nationalities in the race.)

I knew about the legendary "girls of Wellesley College". Everyone in the race did. The students at Wellesley, an all-female college, were the best marathon fans in the world. No words could prepare me for the wave of noise that greeted us from nearly a mile up the road. I chose only to smile and wave at the cheering young women that lined the route. Some of my fellow runners were revelling in the "scream tunnel" experience to a much greater extent. This exuberant show of support helped get me to the half-marathon split in good spirits.

At 1:25 for the half, I was a little ahead of my goal time. Going out too fast was my biggest worry in Boston. After Victoria, I had told myself over and over to not let this happen. Was I headed for trouble? It didn't feel that way, but there were too many unknowns ahead. I pushed aside any thoughts about what this split might mean for my finishing time. One step at a time, I told myself.

The unrelenting downhill course had caused an unusual problem. I must have been braking, enough to cause hot spots on the balls of my feet. Blisters would soon follow. This had never happened to me before. Damn! Just ahead were the infamous hills of Newton, which would hopefully give my feet some relief. First, though, was another mile or more of downhill running into Newton Lower Falls. I decided this would be a poor excuse for a bad performance, so I tried to adjust my footfall to avoid the hot spots.

Then I started to climb. This felt strange after so much descending. I geared down. I felt myself losing some pace through the hills—there are four—although I seemed to be labouring less than many other runners. The carnage began accumulating around me. Some runners were reduced to walking. Others pulled off the road altogether. I found the inner resources to keep moving upward and onward. This was where I expected to reap the rewards for the time and effort I had invested over the past year. I concentrated on the road and nothing else.

Up ahead of me, steps from the crest of the last Newton hill at 20.8 miles, was the true Heartbreak Hill. There, where so many Boston stories tipped towards tragedy, I had a fortuitous moment of inspiration. I spotted Dick Hoyt and his son Rick. The father and son Team Hoyt had tackled innumerable marathons and triathlons, despite Rick being afflicted by cerebral palsy. The family is from the Boston area. In 2001, the Hoyts were competing in the marathon, as they had already done for many years. As usual, Rick was being pushed in a carriage by his father. Their form was unmistakable in silhouette. Framed at the top of the hill, with his head down, I could see how earnestly Dick was working. I passed them at the crest, just as the grade flattened. I gave Dick a pat on the back and wished them both well. The massive crowd that had assembled at this historic and revered location roared its approval as the Hoyts—and I—passed.

For their sake and my own, I was thankful that the course was mainly downhill to the finish. I realized that I could use this chance encounter to motivate myself. It was a good omen for the five miles of racing that remained. I reset myself mentally and did an inventory from head to toe. All told, I was in good shape. My feet had held up pretty well, and the blisters I was worried about never materialized. I felt some irritation on my toes. That was normal. I heard my coach Gord, back on the Lindsay Park track in Calgary, reminding me to relax my shoulders and run tall. The noise from the spectators, now ten-deep on the course, was deafening. Overwhelming. I tumbled through the chaos that had swallowed me up.

I needed to stay disciplined. Steps ahead of a water station, I took the second and last gel from the pocket of my shorts and forced it down. I took in water at every station, despite the cool temperature. Just a gulp and toss the cup away. At the same time, I made sure to keep my feet as dry as possible going through the puddles that had started to form around the water stations.

At about 23 miles, we moved onto Beacon Street, a long stretch with a commuter rail line on our left. I knew this section would be the true test of my aspiration to finish strong. As I had done in previous marathons, I treated myself to short walking breaks through the last several water stations. I knew walking at all was risky—could I start running and get back on form again? Victims of the Newton hills were all around me. The throng lining the road here was unforgiving. Anyone reduced to walking was implored to get running again, and cheered mightily when they did so. Walking or running, all of us moved forward, towards the same goal.

With relief, I caught my first glimpse of the large and iconic CITGO sign that towers over Fenway Park. I recalled the adage that for runners in the marathon the sign seemed to never get any closer. Maybe it was a good thing that the crowds here were so huge and loud. It was a tradition that the Boston Red Sox played a home game on Patriots' Day, and the addition of a stadium full of baseball fans made things even more tumultuous, if that were possible. I searched for the mile markers, little islands of sanity in this crazy river. These became small rewards for my progress.

Amidst the confusion, our procession continued. We were all being drawn by the same magnetic force. I willed myself forward with one thought, that from here the finish line was mere minutes away. Finishing was a sure thing, but just finishing was not the point today. I needed to deliver a performance worthy of this race. I glanced at my watch as I passed the 25-mile banner and for the first time I allowed myself to think of the result that might be possible.

My world shrank to the patch of road directly in front of me. Second by second, I advanced. There was a brief respite from the mayhem after Kenmore Square, as the course dipped through an underpass. The silence itself was shocking. Then, on Commonwealth Avenue, a sharp right-hand turn on a course with almost no turns told me exactly where I was. Hereford Street. I glanced up, to confirm that I could see runners two short blocks ahead of me making a left turn. Yes! It was Boylston Street and the finishing straight. It was so close now. A feeling of joy started to creep into my consciousness.

"Not yet. It's too early," I said, out loud. I could barely hear my own voice. I remembered a trick my high school coach had taught us years before. I locked my gaze onto the lower back of the runner directly in front of me.

Less than a minute later, when I made that final turn, the blue banners marking the finish area came into view. The spectators were already celebrating for me, but I had to get there to make it official. I forgot about my exhausted legs. There was no pain, almost no physical sensation at all. Time slowed down, as this stretch of road seemed to go on forever. And indeed, part of me wanted this feeling not to end. As the finish line came into focus, I reminded myself to soak up everything I could of this experience, this energy, this adulation, in these final metres of the world's greatest marathon. Tears welled in my eyes as I spotted the 26-mile mark. I passed it. Only 385 yards to go—350 metres—less than one lap on a track. Now I could read the numbers on the timing clock. It baited me with the prospect of a finish I had only dared to dream of. I lowered my head, straightened up my form and crossed the line with my arms held high.

The clock read 2:58:56. I had done it. I was a Boston Marathon finisher!

My unsteady walk through the finish area confirmed that I had reached my physical and emotional limit. There was no holding back the torrent now. I was overcome with joy. And relief. I exchanged knowing glances and words of congratulation with other finishers, choking back my emotions in a voice that was no more than a whisper. The amazing volunteers, knowing what this meant to us Boston Marathon finishers, treated us as if we had won the race. When they put my medal around my neck, I *was* a winner. I had joined a very exclusive club.

It was too early to start the post-race analysis, but I knew that the marathon had gone as well as I could have expected. The conditions were excellent. I had managed to avoid any blowups in the punishing second half of the race. I had met my optimistic goal by matching the time I ran in Victoria. I collected my checked bag from the trucks piled high with them, then slowly and gingerly made my way to the rendezvous area beyond the finish, blistered toes throbbing and quads aching, where I met up with Deb and the boys. There, another wave of emotion and exhaustion hit me. They had sacrificed so much to make my dream possible. It was pure joy to see them and begin to share this once-in-a-lifetime experience with them.

The official results package, which arrived in the mail two weeks later, supplied the concrete evidence of my achievement. I had finished in 803rd place among 13,400 finishers, and 174th of more than three thousand in my age group, in the race that runners unanimously held in the highest esteem. The numbers were impressive and satisfying, but they were only numbers. I was at a loss for words to describe what I was feeling. Years later, I still have trouble. It was exceptional. Momentous. *Transcendent.* It was everything I had hoped it would be.

Jolly Old England

TRANSCENDENT OR NOT, I would have very little time to savour my Boston Marathon experience, because my family and I soon embarked on an even bigger adventure: a trans-Atlantic move to England. The idea of a temporary work transfer had been floated some time earlier by my company. We had agreed in principle, but initially our thoughts were directed towards Houston, Texas, where the company had its head office. Through a series of fortuitous events, our destination was changed from Houston to London. That was the good news. Unfortunately, time was not on our side, and for important reasons now long forgotten, our move had to happen in the summer of 2001. There were a thousand details to sort out, and Purvin & Gertz was a small company with none of the resources needed for such a move. We were the only Canadian family they had ever moved to the United Kingdom.

While we managed to get most of the details of our move worked out in the spring of 2001, we secured the necessary UK work visa only a few hours before we boarded the plane in late August. We had decided early in the planning phase of the move to rent our house rather than sell it. There simply was not enough time available for us to put it on the market.

We expected to be in the UK for four years. I would be working in the heart of London. Deb was designated on my work visa as a dependant, which meant she would not be able to work. Our first major decision was to arrange schooling for the boys. We chose to enroll them in an American school. To us, this was a more sensible option than placing them in the much different British system, only to pull them back out when we returned home. The school we chose was in an idyllic setting in Thorpe, a small town in the county of Surrey. Some of the school buildings were five hundred years old. The school catered to the large expatriate community in and around London, meaning that it was expensive. The boys benefited from their time at the school, and Deb and I also made many friends among the cohort of parents.

If we thought we could relax with the boys taken care of, we would have been mistaken. Our main considerations in determining where to live were proximity to the school and the availability of good public transport. We learned how much life in the UK depends on public transportation once I joined the million other commuters who relied on trains and the London Underground—the Tube—to get into Central London each day. My ten-minute commute into downtown Calgary had been laughably easy by comparison. Deb would take on the duties of social convenor and chauffeur-in-chief, doing the school run for the boys and supporting me in my commute.

We endured five weeks of unsettled and unsettling stays in temporary accommodations. We were already feeling homesick when the world was shaken by the terrorist attacks in the US on September 11. That tragic day deeply affected people in Britain and left us, as newcomers, feeling even more disoriented than before. It was a challenging start to this new chapter of our life.

Eventually, thanks to Deb's heroic efforts, we signed a lease on a rental unit in Oldfield Wood, a magnificent gothic-styled complex of renovated townhouses and flats set among beautifully landscaped grounds in Woking, Surrey. Woking was not a quaint English town, but it was close to Guildford and other places with more character. Woking did have one distinct advantage, which was its excellent train connections to London. As was often the case during our time in the UK, serendipity intervened in what had proven to be a difficult search for a suitable place to live. A sympathetic estate agent overheard us explaining our then-desperate plight to his colleague. We had been looking without success, for a furnished house. He suggested that he might know of just the place for us, even though it happened to be unfurnished. He was right.

Oldfield Wood had originally been built as St. Peter's Convent during Victorian times. We moved into unit 20, the former vicarage, a three-storey house adjacent to a small church on the premises. Our house looked out onto a charming courtyard with a fountain. Our neighbours were an eclectic mix of Brits and expatriate families, mainly from Europe but also including some Americans. We were across the courtyard from the parents of Paul Weller, an icon of British pop music. We assumed the role of resident Canadians. As a community, we enjoyed many dinners and social events together. Oldfield Wood was a comfortable walk to the train station in town. Even so, on most days, Deb would drop me off and pick me up, in addition to driving the kids everywhere and back again. She nearly wore out a red Saab 9-3 during our time in England.

My commute was a daily adventure. From Woking, I rode what were called "slam-door trains," odd carryovers from the 1950s with multiple sets of doors on each carriage. The name came from the sound of passengers closing dozens of doors as they got on or off. Once a train got up to speed it was impossible to sit and read, as the harsh suspension would knock its riders around mercilessly.

After surviving the trip to Waterloo Station, I would navigate the labyrinth which was the Tube system. I still recall the unmistakable smell that pervaded the entire system and the pattern on the cloth upholstery of the seats. Why would they use cloth, I wondered? I preferred to stand. On arrival at Green Park station, three levels deep below Piccadilly, I was left with only a ride up the steep and long escalators to reach the welcome fresh air at street level. The trip took forty-five minutes on a good day. Not all days were good.

Our company office was in Mayfair—affluent, upscale Mayfair, with its smart Georgian townhouses, exotic embassies, posh restaurants, and regal parks. The building on Stratton Street was steps from elegant Green Park, which was adjacent to Buckingham Palace. I could see the Ritz Hotel from my second-floor window. The location was as upmarket as they came. Not that our office location mattered much, as our company served clients from all across Europe, the Middle East, Russia and elsewhere.

Once again, I had stepped onto a steep learning curve, which was fine with me. Although the essential aspects of the job were the same as what I had been doing in Calgary for five years—providing technical and commercial advice to clients in relation to their oil, natural gas, or refinery projects—the clients and the office procedures were all new to me. I fit in seamlessly with my office colleagues, some of whom I already knew from previous work projects. Like me, they each faced a daily adventure by commuting into London from different points of the compass. They were a diverse group, and they made me feel welcome right from the beginning.

While we gradually settled into life in the UK, we noticed the many differences from our former life in Canada. Almost everything was different, even if most of the time the distinctions were subtle. We slowly began to learn a whole new vocabulary. We learned that there was such a thing as a TV license, and why we needed one. We experienced the unparalleled, intense frustration that could come from dealing with British banks, government offices and utilities. Doing business with shops was often problematic, too. Why? Well, English society seems to depend on an arbitrary and inflexible system that I dubbed *The Rules*. The Rules were not written down, even though everyone seemed to know and follow them. Assuming our desired outcome of a given interaction to be represented by *X*, where X could be something trivial (like getting a dollop of cream in a coffee, without an extra charge) or significant (like having a credit card approved), I was liable to hear the same phrase.

"Oh no, sir, I could not possibly do—X. The Rules forbid it!"

Coming from Canada, we were amused to see that the English really did not understand winter. Since few drivers had snow tires, a one-inch snowfall in England was enough to shut down the whole country, sometimes for days. It was ironic that the boys had more snow days in England than they ever had back home. One day, in January, we noticed crocuses emerging next to our house. We stood there, staring in amazement for some time, until a neighbour came over and asked if everything was all right.

"Yes. It's just that we wouldn't see these in Calgary for another three months!" Deb said.

One aspect of English life that did seem somehow familiar to me was the prevailing attitude towards alcohol. We observed a much greater incidence of alcohol abuse than we had seen in Canada, particularly among younger people. As newcomers, we theorized about the complex causes of this problem. We began to wonder if it had its roots in a social system that seemed unable to provide ample opportunities for its youth. Naturally my thoughts turned to my father's ongoing challenges with alcoholism, which may have had a historical connection to this part of the world. In the end, we decided it was an issue well beyond our ability to understand.

* * *

I soon turned my mind to how running could be incorporated into our English adventure. As with everything else, there were some differences compared to running in Canada. Right away, I noticed the closer confines of the roadways in England. Everything was narrower and tighter than back home, which meant that cars were often a more present risk factor. By a happy coincidence, there were also many options for running in parks and other public spaces. This always struck me as a paradox. Here was a tiny country, so much more densely populated than western Canada. And yet, there was never a shortage of green spaces to run in.

For our part, Deb and I felt liberated by another difference, and that was the option of running with less clothing on during the milder UK winters. We made a point of running as often as we could without the tights, multiple layers and jackets that would have been essential to survive a winter season in Alberta. Sometimes it was a close call, and we would come home after a damp January run with very pink legs, but it was a joy to even have that choice.

From our house, we had ready access to the Basingstoke Canal. The towpath adjacent to this historic but little-used waterway was a pleasant option for long runs or walks. Woking was situated between the Woodham locks to the east and the Brookwood locks to the west. We would occasionally see a long, narrow canal boat slowly working its way up or down, on its way to we weren't sure where. Carp fishermen sat along the water's edge in the early mornings. Their long poles protruded behind them, leaving us to gingerly step over as we ran by. We never saw anyone catch anything, and given the dark, murky water of the canal we were glad about that.

Woking was a relaxing one-hour run away from the boys' school, when I followed the smaller A and B roads. I would set off from the house early on Saturday mornings, to meet up with Deb and the boys for whatever activities they were involved in. Along the way, I had access to some special places, such as Virginia Water, which was a short distance from Thorpe. A lap around the peaceful lake was about four and a half miles on a shaded gravel path, which made it a fine place to train.

Another of my favourite running locales was Horsell Common, a park that was famous as the landing spot for the Martians in H.G. Wells' classic novel, *War of the Worlds*. Wells had lived in Woking when he wrote the book. We looked for the blue plaque that marked his house. And we were thrilled to learn that our home in Oldfield Wood was integral to his story, because the narrator who gave us details of the horrible destruction wrought by the aliens lived right next door to the convent at the top of Maybury Hill. More serendipity.

I was tempted to try to use my proximity to the lush Royal Parks in London for training, but this was never as easy as I might have hoped. My office had only one small "loo" for the gents, making it difficult, if not downright embarrassing, to change into my running kit. Then, just to reach a bit of green space to run in, I faced the inevitable gauntlet of tourists strolling up and down Piccadilly. And of course, as the offices emptied for people to get a breath of fresh air over lunch, the parks filled up. Under those conditions, running became more trouble than it was worth. Instead, I decided to use my breaks to explore the narrow streets and shopping arcades of Mayfair.

* * *

Amateur clubs were prevalent in the English running community. In Canada, a minority of runners were affiliated with a local running club, whereas running in England was still very much a club-oriented sport. This system seemed like a holdover from a bygone era. It reminded me of the close allegiances the English had to their football clubs, or even to their local pub. England, already geographically tiny compared to Canada, seemed to be quaintly parceled up into even smaller bits.

At the starting line of a local race, I would see singlets from all sorts of running clubs. The local clubs stressed competition, coaching and community. For most amateur athletes, club running was a way to stay involved in the sport after school. In my experience, there was no comparable method of staying with the sport in North America. I thought about my own situation. I had stuck with the sport for years, but almost always as a self-taught runner. I asked myself how much I might have benefitted if a similar system had existed in Canada. I wondered how many of my high school teammates were still actively running and racing.

As an unaffiliated runner in England, I stood out as an exception. When the gun went off at a local race, another thing became clear. Club runners were generally serious runners, and casual runners—joggers, if you like—were less common. In my first 10k race in England, the surge of racers off the start line told me that these runners meant business. I remembered the Around the Bay Race, so many years earlier, when I had been disheartened to line up next to running's hard men. I felt like I had discovered where all those guys had wound up. It was good to be reminded that the competitive environment of serious running still existed. I would have to up my game.

It was no surprise that the English running scene included some eccentric characters. There was the fellow who "ran" the 2002 London Marathon in an antique dive suit that weighed 130 pounds. He finished the race in six days. And Malcolm, the owner of an independent running store near Cranleigh, was an ultrarunner who thought nothing of doing 100-plus-mile races around the English countryside. Malcolm would regale us with tales from his races, like how he would carry Cornish pasties in his shorts for sustenance along the route. We often found ourselves in his store for hours, enchanted by his stories.

* * *

I discovered that as a UK resident, I could parlay my 2001 Boston Marathon performance into a Good for Age entry into the 2003 London Marathon. While I would not say it was a race I had dreamt of running, here was a convenient path to entry. It was a case of now or never, as gaining an entry into this hugely popular race was not easy.

Because the race was a marathon, there would need to be the usual preparations. As luck would have it, one of my office colleagues was an Italian engineer living in England with his family. Roberto was interested in trying the marathon, and he had secured an entry by agreeing to raise money for a charity. This was a big part of the London Marathon experience, and for many people it was their only way in. Hundreds of runners took the opportunity to run the race in a costume—fancy dress, as the English would say. Most of the costumes were much lighter than a dive suit, but some were very elaborate. As if running a marathon were not hard enough!

Roberto and I used our common interest as an excuse to do long runs together in the serene London parks or along the Thames River. He hoped to learn a bit from me about marathon training, and I found our runs to be a convenient way to learn more about the UK. Our family got to know him, his wife, and their young children, and we enjoyed more than one large, authentic Italian meal at their home in Ealing. We were treated like important guests when we visited, and my sons were amused by the dinners that went on for hours.

"Why did you make two roasts *and* pasta?" they would ask our host.

The race itself was somewhat disappointing for both of us. I found several rationalizations for not running as well as I had hoped, none of which was entirely valid. It was true that just getting to the start, by Tube and on foot, had sapped a lot of my energy. It was also true that the racecourse was extremely congested. I was jostled continuously as the multiple starting grids for 33,000 runners were combined into one. During the race, I suffered some blistering due to a poor choice of shoes. Whatever the reasons, I faded badly in the latter stages of the race, losing ten minutes against my goal time. I finished in 3:06. Roberto, who was experiencing the marathon distance for the first time, suffered leg cramps, which hurt his performance. He crossed the line in 3:50, a slower time than he had hoped for.

My initial dissatisfaction with my performance has mellowed with time. In retrospect, I feel that running London was a worthwhile experience. It was a novel way to see other parts of the city and to be part of the annual excuse for a party that Londoners turn the marathon into. If I am totally honest with myself, I must say that my aspirations for going under three hours on the day were unrealistic. Once again, I had to accept my limitations. The lessons were that I should set reasonable expectations, and on some occasions, just live in the moment. After all, I was still a novice when it came to the running scene in England, and we had other priorities as a family during the years we lived there. It was some consolation that I ran a few memorable races during our time in the UK, including an outstanding half marathon in the historic town of Tunbridge Wells.

* * *

We spent our weekends and holidays travelling around the UK and Europe, most of which was within reach of a short drive or flight from our home base in Surrey. It was tempting to try and see everything. Because we knew our time in the country was limited, that was what we tried to do. We wanted to soak up every bit of British society. We drove south to the Isle of Wight and stayed in a lighthouse keeper's cottage. We ventured north to Scotland and stayed in a stately Georgian flat in Edinburgh.

A couple of months before we left England, I tried to make good on a significant oversight by taking the boys to a local football match. With the season winding down, we joined a small, partisan crowd and watched the home side, Woking FC, eke out a 2–1 win in a meaningless game against another fourth division team. Before the match, we loaded up on scarves and other souvenirs, which elicited great excitement in the team shop.

"We have some new supporters!" I heard one volunteer say to her colleague.

I didn't have the heart to tell her we would soon be leaving the country.

I had countless experiences while working in the London office that would not have been possible otherwise. And whether I was travelling for work or pleasure, I already knew that running was the best way to see the highlights of a place I was visiting for the first time. There is no better way to see a city than on foot, so I made it a point to run in each place I visited. I ran along the Black Sea waterfront in the port city of Feodosiya. I jogged through the Old Town in Warsaw, the ancient market in Ankara, and the pedestrian streets of Moscow. I fought the dust and wind during an abbreviated jog from my hotel in Dubai. I had the surreal experience of watching the 2003 World Cycling Championships on television from a hotel room in Bucharest. That year, the road race was held in Hamilton, of all places, so I was delighted to watch the riders traversing the same mountain access roads I knew so well from my youth.

Between work travel and personal trips, I managed to accumulate stamps from twenty-six countries in my passport during the four years we lived in the UK. I established a multitude of new working relationships and broadened my professional experience. As a family, we made friends and collected enough memories to last a lifetime. Our stay was a success in every way.

There were many benefits of living in the UK, and more small annoyances than we could count. On balance, though, I would say that our stay in England was a life-enhancing period for all of us. We grew to love the country, the people, the quirkiness. It was with mixed feelings that we returned home in the summer of 2005. I was more ready than Deb to return to Canada when my work term ended, mainly because I knew bigger professional challenges awaited me back home. And while I was content to return with my fond memories of our time overseas, I was not unhappy to get away from The Rules.

I Won't Be in Here Long, Will I?

JULY 12, 2017 WAS MY SECOND full day in the hospital. It hadn't fully sunk in yet, but there was no denying that I was in Ward 32, at the far end of Unit 100—the stroke unit. After two restless nights and an anxious day, that was about all I knew for certain. One thing was becoming clear—I was luckier than most of the other patients in the unit. Up to this point, at least, I had not suffered any permanent loss of function. The patients around me were not so fortunate. An elderly woman opposite me had had a serious stroke and was debilitated on one side of her body. A young woman diagonally across from me had had a catastrophic cycling accident and had suffered a major stroke as a result. And on my right was a middle-aged woman with various medical issues, in addition to whatever recent events had landed her in the hospital.

I tried not to pay attention to the stories that had intersected with mine, but that was difficult in our close quarters. Fate had brought us together. Conversations from each corner of the ward overlapped one another and betrayed the worry that we were all feeling. The only time I had ever spent in a hospital before was as a visitor, so for me, worry and fear were mixed in equal proportions.

I soon found the pulse of the place. Mornings were when the doctors did their rounds, so depending on what else they were involved with, I could get the feeling of growing anticipation as they worked their way through the unit. After a consultation with the specialist and his inevitable entourage, instructions would be relayed to the unit staff and doctors, so there was not much more that could be done until the next day. That left me to sit in bed, take naps, plan for meals, and take more walks. For the time being, I was taking aspirin and Plavix, the antiplatelet drugs I had been on since my first visit to the ER. It seemed that the doctors were leaning towards continuation of this program. But the plan was far from finalized, given the unusual nature of my case.

I think it was for exactly that reason that I found myself standing at a computer screen in the nursing station, discussing my situation with Dr. Demchuk. I regretted my initial brusqueness with him, and I told him so. I also told him I was curious to know more about my medical condition. In what was to become our common practice throughout my hospital stay, we talked candidly about my test results and my treatment. He called up pictures from my CT scans and my first MRI. Between us, there was a lot of pointing at test results on the screen and animated gestures to the back of my head.

The CT scans had networks of white lines on a black background, which looked like roads on a map. These were the major arteries in my neck and head. Dr. Demchuk showed me a little black gap in one of the lines, which indicated the spot where my left vertebral artery was blocked. It was just at the point where that artery branched up at right angles from the subclavian artery. He explained that whereas the first scan had shown that my left vertebral artery was partially blocked a few days earlier, the second scan showed it being completely blocked. I now had a proximal occlusion of the left vertebral artery—the word *near* had been dropped.

Then Dr. Demchuk showed me the pictures of my brain from the MRI.

"See those white dots? They're dead spots in your brain. I'm ninety percent sure they are embolisms, resulting from clots originating at the blockage in your vertebral artery."

I didn't understand what the doctor was telling me, and I asked him to back up a bit. He explained that there are two types of strokes. An embolic stroke is caused by a blood clot that has broken off from another location in the body and travelled through the bloodstream to lodge in a blood vessel. A hemorrhagic stroke happens when a blood vessel bursts, causing bleeding in the brain.

I could tell that Dr. Demchuk found my case interesting. He asked about my habits and family history. He was curious about my long connection to running. Perhaps he was looking for clues about the cause of my arterial blockage. Dr. Demchuk asked what I did for a living. I told him that I was a chemical engineer and I explained that throughout my career I had dealt mainly with oil refineries, which rely on the transfer of fluids in pipes. When I told him that I worked at the National Energy Board, the agency responsible for regulating Canada's energy pipelines, we both immediately saw the irony—here was a pipeline engineer having problems with his arteries. That became an inside joke for us. The bottom line was that he could see I was familiar with the flow of liquids in pipes. I got it when we talked about arterial blood flow.

He mused that it probably would be a good idea for us to consider an angiogram. He told me that this would be an invasive procedure, with its own risk of causing a stroke. One chance in two hundred, he guessed. However, he thought that it would be worth taking that risk, because the results would shed light on what was really happening with my arteries. He called another doctor, and I overheard them talking about the pros and cons of going ahead. Despite the inherent risk from the angiogram, they agreed it would be beneficial. The procedure would be scheduled sometime over the next day or two, subject to availability of the equipment.

I took the opportunity to ask him a question I had been afraid to ask up to that point.

"What is the worst-case scenario? I mean, what could happen to me?"

Dr. Demchuk paused before answering. "That would be a massive basilar stroke. You would basically be a vegetable. Mind you, that is a really low-probability event."

Low probability or not, I felt my knees buckle as I realized it was me that we were talking about. It was all too much.

* * *

In the early hours of July 14, after an unstable trip to the bathroom, I was lying awake in bed. I felt dizzy and was close to losing consciousness. The room was spinning. I heard a television set that one of my neighbours had left on, just as she had done the night before. Then, I was so bothered by the television that I rang the nursing station and asked them to shut it off. But this time, the sound was distant. It swirled around me like the noise of the spectators at the race in May. Maybe I had another episode of vertigo, different only in that I was half asleep. I felt as if I was floating in water and being pulled around by the currents. I clung to the TV broadcast, with the words as my life preserver. I told myself that if I could keep listening to the television, I would be okay. This feeling continued for an uncertain time. I drifted off.

I somehow made it through the night, still feeling off. I let the nurses know that I had had a bad night, although I had trouble explaining just what was wrong. I was still feeling dizzy and off-balance, but I managed to get up for the bathroom. As soon as I got back into bed, I had another episode of screeching in my ears, and then my eyes went out of control. It was exactly like the TIA I'd had on the treadmill. The current one lasted no more than a minute.

A little later, a nurse came by to tell me that an appointment had been arranged for an angiogram that morning. On my own, I walked into the hallway, where a porter had parked a gurney. We waited there together for a little while. Eventually, I got bumped from the procedure due to a more urgent case. I returned to bed under my own steam, even though I was still somewhat unstable on my feet.

I got back into bed and looked up at the television set. Almost immediately, a black curtain was pulled across my right eye by an invisible hand. It stopped exactly halfway into my field of vision. I could not see the right side of the screen. I couldn't even see my right hand. In a growing panic, I pushed the call button for help. Peter, a young nurse practitioner whom I had come to know, quickly arrived to look at me. By now, I was familiar with the battery of tests that are used to check stroke symptoms, so I anticipated the one in which he held up a different number of fingers on each hand. I instinctively cheated by turning my head to see the right side. This was a trick Peter had seen before. I had to admit to him that I couldn't see from my right side at all. My breath shortened as I grew more frantic. Peter tried to calm me down and reassured me that the doctor would soon be there. After a short time, maybe five minutes, the black curtain slowly retreated to the place in my brain from where it originated. I could see from both eyes again.

* * *

The blockage in my left vertebral artery, just as it branched north from the subclavian artery and towards my brain, had probably been there and growing for some time. The first, and maybe the best, answer the doctors could give me was that my condition was likely due to genetics. It may have been due to arterial damage that I had sustained at some time in the past. Or there may have been another explanation.

Regardless of its cause, there seemed to be a consensus that there was little I could have done to prevent the blockage from forming, especially given my healthy lifestyle. The blockage had not just happened in the weeks prior to my admission to the hospital. It seemed that only when the last bit of the artery was being affected, did I start experiencing symptoms like the prism in my vision or the spells of vertigo.

As for what could be done to address my condition, it basically came down to three options: to treat it with medication (to stop any further blockages from forming), to put in a stent to open the artery (to do an intervention, in the euphemistic language of the doctors), or to operate to do a bypass around the blockage. Several days into my hospital stay, I was told that the medication option was the preferred approach, although Dr. Demchuk confided that he was still discussing my case with an intervention specialist. As for the surgical option, that might have been a challenge for the doctors in Calgary.

"If you lived in certain large cities in the United States, you'd have had the surgery by now," Dr. Demchuk told me. "And if we do decide to go that route, we'd probably look to send you to the States to have it done."

Dr. Demchuk and his colleague, Dr. Menon, were surprisingly candid when discussing treatment options with us. I came to appreciate their candour. Knowing how busy they were, seeing to the needs of their many patients, I was thankful for every minute I got with them. The neurologists found my case intriguing. After all, I was not their typical patient. I secretly wished I could be a bit less special.

* * *

The stroke events of July 14 shook me to my core. I felt my situation suddenly becoming more precarious. My somewhat cavalier attitude towards my condition, and my impatience with the medical process I was caught up in, gave way to a darker perspective. This was serious.

My latest TIAs had indicated to the doctors that a mild treatment program was not working, so Dr. Menon ordered me to be hooked up to an intravenous drip of heparin, a strong anticoagulation drug. Heparin replaced the aspirin I had been taking. They gave me an initial strong dose and started monitoring my blood for its effectiveness. This meant running blood tests in the lab every six hours, as the doctors zeroed in on the optimal anticoagulation target. Events has taken another unexpected and frightening turn. Discussions about when I could go home were pushed off the agenda. Getting control of my symptoms became our primary objective.

The TIAs in the morning were only the beginning of a busy day. After the start of my heparin drip, a spot opened for me to have an angiogram in the afternoon. On the long gurney ride to the clinic, I had another chance encounter that left a lasting impression on me. I met a young porter whom I would see a few times during my time at Foothills. Dean and I started chatting, and soon we were like old buddies. I was happy to have someone take my mind off what had happened earlier that day. Dean was an avid fan of classic rock, and by the time he had navigated us through the labyrinth of the hospital complex to our destination, we had touched on Pink Floyd, Led Zeppelin, his favourite Rush concerts, and even his coincidental connection to Hamilton—he had once travelled there with his band. It was just the diversion I needed.

As Deb and I waited outside the diagnostic imaging clinic, we talked with the impossibly young but highly competent doctor who would perform the procedure. I had no idea what to expect, and I was worried. Dr. Al-Qahtani did much to reassure me. I could scarcely believe the size of the equipment in the operating theatre. The nurses and technicians were so calm and professional that I put myself completely in their hands. I had no other choice.

The angiogram procedure involved inserting a probe into my groin and up towards my heart. The injection of dye would allow video to be taken of the vascular system in my neck and head. Everything went well, and the procedure was over quite quickly. Deb told me she was able to watch the results on a large screen as the procedure was being done. It seemed out of this world when she described the video images of blood flowing into and out of my brain. It is not something you ever expect to see. Later, my curiosity got the better of me, and I asked to see the video for myself.

I returned to the stroke unit, but only briefly, because another MRI had been scheduled for later in the day. After the angiogram, I had to lie still without moving my right leg for about six hours, to avoid damaging the injection site. That was more difficult than the MRI procedure itself. Lying absolutely still in the MRI machine was the most uncomfortable and claustrophobic experience I'd had since being admitted. By the end, my leg and my back were screaming. Added to that, the noise and close quarters of the MRI were almost unbearable. I concentrated on my breathing, imagining myself out for a pleasant run along the Elbow River, as I waited for the torture to be over.

That night, I fell into a fitful sleep. I struggled to get comfortable, while not moving my right leg. Meanwhile, lab technicians showed up every few hours to take a blood sample for a check on my heparin dose. One of the techs inadvertently ripped a patch of skin off my elbow when removing the tape from an earlier sample. I screamed in pain. Somewhere in my foggy memory, a young doctor stopped by to wake me, and to explain that the MRI has shown them that yes, more damage had been done by the latest TIAS. More white spots.

I felt like I was at the bottom of a deep pit, with no way to get out.

* * *

The next day, things seemed to have improved. My attitude was more positive than the events of the previous day would justify. I couldn't explain why that should be, but I attributed it to having a number of visitors during the day. Whatever I had gone through, I kept reminding myself that I was in good hands.

I resigned myself to my new routine, pushing my IV drip around with me. I forced myself to get up for the bathroom, despite the discomfort at the angiogram site. Even without the tangible proof of the MRI results, I knew that the previous day's TIAS had done some damage. Although the doctor had suggested that the damage was in the part of the brain dealing with vision, which would make sense given my episode with the black curtain, I did not notice any lasting changes there. What I did notice was that I was less stable on my feet than I had been before. I was relieved to have an IV pole to hang on to for balance. I could only hope that the damage would not be permanent.

The shift nurse moved me from my location in the most distant ward to a small, isolated room next to the nursing station. After the change in my circumstances, with the recent TIAS, and knowing that I would need to be monitored for a couple of days after the angiogram, they wanted to have me closer to hand. My new location in room 35 could be closed off from the noise of the wards, so I managed to sleep a little better than I had until then.

I tried to get my mind off my situation with an iPod and some tunes. The tactic worked, but only to an extent, and that seemed to confirm that I was an emotional wreck. Without warning, I burst into tears when I heard Chris Martin of Coldplay describe what it meant to contemplate a future with a significant loss, in the song *Fix You*: "And the tears come streaming down your face, when you lose something you can't replace." He was singing about lost love, but for me it was an altogether different thing that I could not stand to lose. The feeling of loss started with the loss of competitive running, but maybe it was really much more than that—loss of my former self.

After a day or two of uncertainty, on July 17, Deb suggested that we go for a walk beyond the confines of the tenth floor. We had seen everything in the immediate vicinity of my bed anyway. The angiogram incision was feeling better and I knew that walking would be good for me. But I hesitated.

"What if I see someone I know?" I asked.

"Who are you going to see?" she replied. "Let's go."

So, with the permission of the unfailingly helpful nurses, we headed for the elevator.

"I'm not sure about this," I said, as we waited for the slow ride down.

"Don't worry. No one will see you," Deb reassured me.

The elevator doors opened onto the busy main floor lobby, and we cautiously stepped out. I looked up to meet the eyes of Dr. Stephen Wood, a friend and long-time running colleague from Adrenaline Rush and a doctor at Foothills. We had run together in the K-100 Relay three weeks earlier. His gaze said it all, as he looked me up and down in my hospital garb, complete with IV.

"What the heck happened to you—?" he asked.

I felt my face turn red with embarrassment. I shot a quick look at Deb, an I-told-you-so kind of look. But by then, there was nothing to be done. I explained, for the first of many times, what had transpired over the last couple of weeks, what had brought me to the hospital, and more specifically, what had brought me to the tenth-floor stroke unit. Stephen was in a hurry with his own responsibilities, but he promised to come and visit me.

I soon came to realize that this chance meeting, the one that I had expressed concern to Deb about, was the best thing that could have happened to me. Stephen was a generous and caring friend as I grappled with the uncertainty and the fear about my predicament. He visited me almost every day for the rest of my hospital stay. He listened to the specialists as we discussed treatment, and most important of all, he gave me his own take on the options that were being tossed around. As much as I had felt lost at sea in my dream a few nights earlier, now I felt I had managed to get myself back on solid ground.

On the question of treatment options, Stephen ventured an opinion that helped me put things into perspective. He reminded me that I had had no symptoms since starting on heparin. The fact I could function more or less normally seemed to confirm I had adequate collateral blood flow. But more to the point, he felt that to consider any kind of intervention or surgery was to introduce significant risks associated with procedures in and around the neck. He rhymed off a list of possible complications for me to think about. I saw his point.

Deb and I ventured a little further afield. On the evening of July 18, she proposed that we take a walk outside. It was stifling hot, and Calgary was being blanketed by smoke from forest fires in British Columbia. We slowly made our way to a viewpoint on the south side of the hospital, a spot that overlooked the hill that Mahedi and I had been training on just days earlier. It was the hill workout we had willingly cut short because we were still feeling the effects of the K-100 Relay. Except now, I was wearing a hospital gown instead of my running gear.

We sat on a bench and surveyed the hazy scene in front of us.

The sun had been replaced by an angry red blob in the sky. I had an ominous thought.

"I don't want this to be our last walk together," I said, through the tears that began to well up in my eyes.

"It won't be," she promised.

From where we were sitting, we could see the bluff on the south side of the Bow River, where the Douglas Fir Trail traverses from Edworthy Park to the Crowchild Bridge. It is a strenuous path that goes steeply up one side of the escarpment, and then steeply back down. Deb had always been curious about it but had never seen it. I had run it dozens of times with Rob, my friend from Shell, and I often used it as a test of my fitness when I was getting close to a goal race. That seemed a lifetime ago. We agreed to hike the route as soon as I was able. I wondered in silence how long that would be, if ever.

The focus of our daily discussions with the doctors turned to an exit strategy from the hospital. Since it was not feasible to stay indefinitely on a heparin IV, they explained that it would be necessary to transition me to a pill form of the same drug. This is warfarin. Although the transition is relatively straightforward, it would take a few days to accomplish, since it involves adding warfarin—up to an appropriate dosage—and then cutting off the heparin. I was already feeling like a pin cushion, so what was a bit more poking?

The objective with any of the conventional anticoagulants, which are often colloquially called blood thinners, is to maintain a target efficacy. This is determined, through frequent blood tests, by the International Normalized Ratio, or INR. The INR is a standardized measure of clotting time for a person's blood while on the anticoagulant, relative to clotting time for a person not on the drug. Simple to say, but sometimes not so simple to accomplish. And as I learned from a Google search, warfarin has a reputation of being hard to control, because its effectiveness as an anticoagulant can be affected by diet, interactions with other medications and many other variables. How often I would need an INR test would be decided in due course.

The process started smoothly, and my INR began responding to the warfarin. I continued with the other drugs and added a dose of Tylenol for a pain in my left shoulder. This was new. The shoulder pain intensified as the pain in my groin from the angiogram receded. Although I raised the question of whether and how this shoulder pain might be connected to my underlying issue—the blocked left vertebral artery—the usual response was a shrug of the shoulders and an offer of more Tylenol. Staff in the unit had more pressing issues to deal with.

By then, Deb and I knew many of the nurses and other staff. They got to know us too. One of the orderlies checked on me regularly and kept me well supplied with heat packs and extra desserts. The nurses stopped asking if I was okay when the machine that checked my vital signs alerted them to my low heart rate. "Oh right, you're the runner," they would say. Deb found her way around the unit and would grab me a warm blanket if I needed one, rather than bothering anyone else.

We did as much walking as possible. We saw everything there was to see on the tenth floor and ventured outside when I felt up to it. The walking helped to clear the bruising from the angiogram. My INR results slowly climbed toward the target range that the doctors had in mind. Meanwhile, I had been moved again, this time to another of the wards in the unit. This one, Ward 36, was a busy place, close to the nursing station and noisy. Getting a good night's sleep was out of the question. I settled for afternoon naps, which I began to look forward to.

I had a steady stream of visitors. Our son Matt joined Deb during her daily visits, even though he was busy with a new job. He was considerate enough to bring in a cribbage board and despite my condition, not considerate enough to let me win. Several of my running buddies and my office colleagues dropped in to see me. Phil was generous with his time, and he checked in on me frequently. Not many people in the office were aware of my situation, but as I saw from the emails and texts that had started coming in, word had gotten out that I was having some health problems. I also got regular calls from Mom and Kathleen. It was nice to know that people were worried about me. Even so, I felt like I was watching life drift slowly past me.

By the morning of July 20, my INR level had reached the target range, and discussion in the morning rounds turned to my discharge. It had been almost a week since my last round of symptoms. I took the opportunity to share my concerns with Dr. Menon about the sustainability of a plan based only on medication. He again expressed his confidence in the strategy.

Dr. Menon ordered my heparin drip to be disconnected around noon. Later, as a precursor to going home, I met with physical therapists to discuss my condition. They watched me walk up and down the hall and navigate a flight of stairs. After a restful nap, I had another visit from my office colleagues. We laughed and talked about my imminent return to the office. Deb came in and ate dinner with me. We went for a walk outside, and we admired the beautiful scene from the hilltop. The haze from the forest fires had dissipated—it was a lovely evening. I felt liberated, not having an IV pole with me. We discussed changes to our fall vacation plans, since I would not be able to fly for a while. Rather than going away, we decided we could do things closer to home, like take in the Calgary International Film Festival and visit the Glenbow Museum. It was an ideal evening, full of optimism.

The night of July 20 changed everyone's plans for me—yet again.

At about 2 A.M., a lab technician came to take a blood sample. I got up shortly after to take a pee. As soon as I got back into bed, I had another TIA. It started like the previous ones, with loud ringing in my ears. I pushed the call button for the nurse, but when I tried to speak, I could not make my mouth form the words. My tongue was a frozen lump. Then my arms started moving on their own. They were jerky and spasmodic. These were new and different symptoms from the ones I had experienced before. I felt a rising panic.

The duty nurse arrived within a couple of minutes. By then, the worst of the TIA was over, and I was able to speak again. My voice was a slurred mumble. I had also regained control of my arms. The uncontrolled movements had been replaced by a general feeling of numbness. Although I was confused and sluggish, I could understand what was going on, and I could still complete all the usual stroke tests that the nurse put me through.

The nurse contacted the neurology resident, who ordered an immediate CT scan. Another scan meant another dose of radiation, but I was in no mood to debate the issue. As I waited on the gurney for the scan, the resident arrived to see me. It was Andrea, the same young doctor who had admitted me more than a week earlier. I babbled something to her about being scared and not understanding what had just happened to me.

"Don't worry," she said. "We'll know more when we look at the scan."

I needed to see Deb. When the scan was finished, and they returned me to the tenth floor, I called her and tried to explain what had happened. I was rambling incoherently. She could tell I was in a panic and she let me know she would see me soon.

Although it lasted only a few minutes, this TIA shook me more than the previous ones. I could still feel the residual impacts, specifically in my left hand, which was weaker and slower than my right. My balance was thrown off, but my eyesight and hearing seemed not to have been affected.

I had limited interaction with the doctors the following day because they were attending to serious issues with other patients. Nevertheless, Dr. Demchuk ordered more tests. One test used Doppler radar to measure blood flow in the cerebral arteries. A contraption was screwed onto my head that looked suspiciously like Dr. Emmett Brown's brain-wave analyzer in the movie *Back to the Future*. The test took about an hour, during which I was not to move or talk. That was okay with me, since I did not feel much like moving or talking anyway.

Dr. Demchuk had also ordered another MRI test, my third. While I waited to be called for that, the doctors hooked me up with a Holter monitor, a portable electrocardiogram machine that measures electrical activity in the heart. I would have to wear it for a day or so. The doctors wanted to check, again, to see if my heart might have been the source of my latest ischemic attack.

It was impossible to get any rest in the ward. Next to me was an older man who spent all his time trying to escape. He had a dangerous fall next to my bed. From then on, he was restrained, but still managed to rip out his IV twice. The fellow diagonally across from me rang for the nurses at least once every minute. His requests included, but were not limited to, his wallet, the telephone, his watch, different food, his book, the remote control, his pants, and most often, warm blankets. He asked for so many that it had become something of a joke among the staff.

"Nurse, I need another warm blanket," I heard him ask for the hundredth time.

"No Henry, we need some for the rest of the hospital," came the reply.

Good for you, I thought. The people working here are heroes.

I was summoned for the MRI early on Saturday morning, after a terrible night of listening to Henry. The previous MRI tests were unbearably noisy and claustrophobic. This time, given the current situation in my room, I looked forward to having the test as a welcome break for an hour.

Given his heavy workload, Dr. Demchuk had committed to review the test results with Deb and me over the weekend. I agreed, since I was apparently going to be there for a few more days and my schedule was wide open. I watched the British Open on television, guilt-free, while I waited to see him. I felt strangely confident when we did sit down, but that didn't last long. He told us that the Doppler test had shown what he considered to be satisfactory blood flow in my vertebral arteries. That was one bit of good news. However, the MRI test had revealed what he described as a close call. He told us that the TIA had been from an embolism that had just missed the hypothalamus, the brain's control centre. It had also left a blockage in another cerebral artery. He explained how this might account for my latest symptoms. I felt myself swoon again.

Despite this negative news, Dr. Demchuk reassured us that he did not consider the latest TIA as a failure of the medication. In fact, he believed this was still the preferred option. He went so far as to predict we would be sipping a scotch together in six months. He said that he would continue to confer with the other specialists and give us their best recommendation in a couple of days. While they had been open about including me in their discussions up to that point, he did make it clear that I was to be left out of the loop for now. He didn't need to say more, but I knew why. They might say things that I would not want to hear.

* * *

Of all the tests I had during my hospital stay, the angiogram of my brain was the most revealing. I think this was Dr. Demchuk's hope when he ordered the test. It was self-evident that I could stand and walk and see straight. This confirmed that blood was getting into my brain, even with a compromised left vertebral artery. The angiogram showed in real time how this was happening.

When I mustered the courage to ask Dr. Demchuk to show me the video, it was an odd and fascinating experience. How strange it was to watch a video of the blood flow in my own brain. It would certainly qualify as a type of out-of-body experience. The video provided proof that my body had adapted to the progressively blocked left vertebral artery. I had what is called collateral artery development, which meant that my body had built new blood vessels around the blockage.

The video showed a dark segment just above the subclavian artery—the now fully-blocked part of the artery, where no blood was passing. Above that, feathery arteries progressively filled with blood—one, two, three—after each beat of my heart, then filled the larger vertebral. Almost immediately the blood was gone, as the vertebral artery pushed it up into my brain. A second later, the cycle repeated itself. This improvised system was working, somehow. I could only stare in disbelief.

When I got over my initial shock, my chemical engineer's mind picked up on another thing I saw in the angiogram. The video showed a segment of the vertebral artery, the short piece between the blockage and the first collateral connection, that piping experts would call a *dead leg*. As the collateral arteries did their job, filling the vertebral on every pulse so that blood could be delivered to its final destination, some blood filled the non-functional part of the artery, just below the collaterals. I tried to estimate how long this dead leg was—probably not more than a centimetre.

Dr. Demchuk and I had very different areas of expertise, but we both came to the same conclusion as we looked at the video of blood flowing into and out of this compromised vertebral artery. To a chemical engineer, having a dead leg in a piping system is not an effective design.

"This isn't how anyone would design a piping system," I told him.

A neurologist would agree with that opinion, but for a different reason. The presence of a dead leg meant an increased risk of blood clots. The possibility of blood pooling in this small segment of the artery—the stump, if you like—meant that the blood would stagnate. Stagnant blood creates a risk of clot formation, which could then be transmitted up into my brain.

Dr. Demchuk explained that this was the same phenomenon that occurred in people with atrial fibrillation, where the heart's pumping rhythm got out of sequence, leading to pooling and the formation of blood clots in the upper chambers of the heart. Anytime clots are being formed in the body, there is an increased risk of stroke, as the clots move through the arteries. This is called an embolism. I understood then why the doctors had ordered an echocardiogram of my heart soon after I was admitted. They wanted to satisfy themselves that my heart was not the source of my strokes. I could also see why blood thinning medication made sense, to stop the formation of clots in my vertebral artery.

I had some answers but many more questions. Where did those collateral arteries come from? How long did they take to develop? How reliable were they? The doctors were able to provide some answers, based on their experience with other patients. What seemed clear was that the collateral development had taken place over quite a period of time.

I shuddered as I realized that I was staring at an explanation for the pain I had experienced on the left side of my neck and my left shoulder in the past. As it happened, for much of the time between 2010 and 2012, I had suffered from severe pain in exactly the same location—my left shoulder and the lower part of my neck. It was particularly bad during long runs and strenuous workouts and seriously hindered my preparation for a couple of marathons, including the 2011 Boston Marathon. I will likely never know for sure, but I believe that is when I was calling those secondary blood vessels into action. It all made sense.

I explained my theory to the doctors, but they avoided saying much about whether it was correct. We certainly couldn't prove it. The fact was that my body appeared to have figured out that there was a need to increase the blood supply to my brain. It had responded, perhaps years earlier, by growing new arterial connections to my left vertebral artery. I was awestruck by the thought that my body was capable of this type of adaptation. It seemed so unlikely as to be impossible. I was lucky to still be alive, and it would seem I had running to thank for it.

* * *

The close call that Dr. Demchuk described had done some damage. This became clear when Deb and I ventured outside for our short walks around the perimeter of the hospital. In what would become the most lasting physical reminder of my TIAs, my balance was impaired when standing or walking. It was as if someone were grabbing me by the scruff of the neck and the belt and pitching me forward. I was left feeling lightheaded and dizzy and my limbs were lethargic. As a result, our walks began to be punctuated by frequent stops, because I needed to sit or lean on something until the feeling passed.

I tried not to think about what another TIA might do.

Return to Life ... And Death

AS WE ALLOWED TIME FOR our family to transition back to Canadian life, and for me to take on an expanding role in my company, I found that 2006 and 2007 were occupied with many other things besides running. My first objective was to renew client relationships after four years overseas, which took a lot of my time. I had assumed the role of office manager when we returned to Calgary, which meant that I was responsible for the thousand details that came with the job. I learned immediately that managing a diverse group of people, even people I knew well, would be more demanding than dealing with the technical issues I was familiar with. All at once, everyone's problems had become my problems. I decided I should rely on the same principles that had worked for me as a parent for eighteen years, along with a healthy dose of common sense.

The boys, too, were making their own transitions back to life in Canada. Matt started university in Vancouver, which meant a move even farther west for him. That would not have happened without Deb's doing the bulk of the organizing. Daniel started high school in Calgary. Simultaneously, he and Deb took the initial steps onto a path that was to become a big part of our lives—aviation. At Daniel's insistence, they looked into private pilot training— "you can start as early as fourteen," he had informed us—and soon they had both signed up for ground school at the busy Springbank Airport, west of the city. Her logic, which was infallible, went like this: since he was too young to drive himself to the lessons, she might as well start the training too. This would eventually lead to career paths for both of them in the aviation industry. A small part of me was jealous, but I already had more on my plate than I could handle.

With all of that to keep us occupied, it was 2008 before my thoughts could turn again to my old companion, running. Twenty years after my first experience in the Jasper–Banff Relay, and as proof that it really is a small world, or at least a small Calgary running community, I had a chance to run in the revamped relay. The race had been relaunched as the Banff–Jasper Relay and was now organized in two phases, north and south. Starts for each phase were simultaneous, which meant that the race could be completed during daylight hours. I thought back to my adventures with night stages in the original relay and decided I could do without that kind of excitement.

My good friend Mahedi, the same friend who had been such a wonderful partner for interval training years earlier, and who would come back into my life before and during my hospitalization, had approached me in the spring of 2008 about running on a team organized by none other than Janice McCaffrey. Her team was called Adrenaline Rush, and she had recently begun coaching a club with the same name. Mahedi put forward my name, knowing that Janice needed a couple of spare runners.

I was coincidentally going to be in Jasper for a conference the weekend of the race, so it would be convenient for me to join up with the team there. Deb and I marvelled at the majestic sights along the Icefields Parkway, a drive we had not done for many years. Despite my lack of race fitness, I ran the second-to-last stage into Jasper, on the northern leg of the race. I handed off to Mahedi for the last stage. It was a nice bit of closure. We did well, finishing second in the open division. It was just like old times. In an ironic twist nine years later, Janice would again need spares for a relay team, and I would be the one to put Mahedi's name forward.

This race was my first direct encounter with Janice. She was an accomplished race walker, and a three-time Olympian. I had seen her at local races for many years. Although I hadn't met her before the Banff–Jasper outing, I certainly knew her by reputation. This was the beginning of a long and fruitful relationship.

* * *

During this period, but really since we had moved away from Ontario, Dad's health continued to deteriorate. I would have trouble putting too precise a timeline on things. There was a straight line between his drinking and his declining health. I'm not sure the details really matter. Aside from the impact of falls and other mishaps, which might have been expected for someone in the throes of alcoholism, he began to deteriorate in more serious ways.

He contracted Chronic Lymphocytic Leukemia, or CLL, a form of cancer that starts in blood stem cells and develops slowly over months or years. It is a disease that can be treated in various ways, but I don't think Dad was really interested in any extraordinary measures. He had a fatalistic view of life, and probably would have made a joke about it, no doubt something about leaving him out with the trash when he died. His treatment program for CLL involved monitoring the progress of the disease and dealing with the complications that it caused. He received regular intravenous immune globulin injections at the cancer hospital in Hamilton. This therapy is used for those CLL patients who don't produce enough antibodies to fight infections. It was a chore for my mother to get him to the hospital, wait several hours for the treatment to be done, and then get him back home. This regimen went on for several years.

His diet, mainly comprising alcohol, was deficient in many ways. He contracted a form of dementia common among alcoholics, which is caused by a severe deficiency of thiamine, or vitamin B1. As a result of this deficiency, he started having problems with memory, movement, vision and coordination.

It became abundantly clear that the only recourse for my long-suffering mother was to have Dad committed to a long-term care facility. This decision caused her untold anguish, but it was the only feasible option. He could no longer take care of himself. He was losing his mind and he was physically deteriorating. Of course, he would not or maybe could not, stop drinking. Mom could not restrain him, so he would find his way to any of a number of watering holes near the house. The situation had become untenable.

After several emergency room visits, Dad was moved in 2002 to a facility called Victoria Gardens, not far from the house. For once and for all, his drinking stopped. The abrupt end to a lifetime of alcohol abuse was, I suppose, not much different than it would be for a drug addict. The process of drying out was likely as hard on Mom as it was on Dad. We were living in England at the time, so we were insulated from the whole process. Eventually, though, Dad did begin to respond in a positive way to the move. His condition stabilized, and his mind cleared a little. The damage was irreversible, but at least some of his symptoms were eased by a better diet and the attention of his caregivers.

On top of everything else, Dad contracted shingles. He was seriously debilitated by the disease, which caused significant nerve damage in his right hand. For months afterwards, Mom would urge him to do physiotherapy, to squeeze a ball or exercise his arm to regain more function. It was a futile effort because he seemed to have little interest in helping himself. Instead, the loss of most of the use of his hand further compounded his decline.

I visited him whenever I was back in Hamilton. I would go with Mom to see him. In his prime, Dad had been fond of vigorous walking, and thought nothing of walking downtown from our house, a distance of about three miles. It had been a point of pride for him that he did not need a car to get around. He walked everywhere. Now, that robust man was gone. He had been replaced by an old man, who could only shuffle as far as the sunroom at the end of the corridor. His hand had been rendered nearly useless by his bout of shingles. His mind was clouded by dementia. Seeing how he was after stabilizing in his current situation, I could only imagine how he had been at the depths of his decline.

But occasionally there would be a flash of his sharp wit, or he would toss out a word to solve a crossword clue. Somewhere beneath the damage in his brain he still had a place for the kind of trivia that had always been his forte. It was the same when I watched him carry on with the staff. I could tell that the men and women who cared for him had fallen for his charm. It was reminiscent of the days when I would see him at work in Hamilton's main post office.

As a small kid, I knew that my father was important. The lobby of the building where he worked was beautiful, clad with pink and grey marble, and finished with heavy brass railings. Mom would sometimes take us inside if she had to meet him for something. We would look for Dad behind one of the impressive brass windows they called the wickets. It never occurred to me to ask why a man who sold stamps and money orders for a living should be important. To me, and apparently to his customers, he was. His casual banter showed how much he loved working with the public. It was the same when he was with his friends, or when the family was together for an important event, but only in that narrow window between his being sober and having had too many drinks. At those times, at his most personable, I wanted to be just like him.

I had trouble reconciling the differences between those versions of my father and the man sitting in front of me in this nursing home. One scene sticks with me. Mom, Dad and I were sitting in the sunroom, working on a crossword. By then his contributions were offered in a voice that was little more than a whisper. As we sat and visited, idly passing time as we filled in our puzzle, one of the health aides came in and asked if Dad needed anything. Was it time for a haircut? Mom said no, that he was probably okay.

"What about his nails?" he asked.

I had to stop, because it wasn't clear what he meant. Then I realized that he was offering to tend to Dad's toenails. Mom said yes. So, I watched, in a bit of shock, as the healthcare worker took care of this small task. It dawned on me that neither he nor my mother would have been able to do it. I knew he could never leave this place.

Dad's room was on the second floor of the facility and overlooked the walkway to the front door. It was our custom to wave to him on our way out. As I looked up at him and waved on that day, I had a strange feeling that he may not be with us much longer. This might be the last time I would see him. It turned out my premonition was right.

He died of a heart attack shortly after my visit. It was the Thanksgiving weekend in October 2009. He was seventy-five. When Paul called to tell me the news, my first reaction was to go out and run one of my favourite routes, so I could have my father in my thoughts for a few quiet minutes. He was a decent man and a good father, and I had much to thank him for. Still, I grappled with my feelings for a man who had serious failings. Coming to terms with my feelings about him would take time.

* * *

Running in the 2008 Banff–Jasper Relay had once again revived my interest in serious training. I needed a goal. I had kept myself motivated by racing the occasional 10k or half marathon, knowing that it was important to do more than aimless running. During my long runs on Sunday mornings with a few old friends, I learned that several of them had joined the Adrenaline Rush club. They all spoke highly of Janice and her training program. My first objective had to be to get back into reasonable shape. To that end, I knew I needed to incorporate interval training into my regimen. I had not run intervals regularly since Mahedi coached us on the Talisman Centre track, before our move to England.

As it had done a number of times in the past, the marathon was beckoning again. I was considering a return to Boston in 2011, but I was of two minds about going back. It had been nearly ten years since my first Boston experience, and I knew it would be impossible to duplicate the positive feelings I still had from that race. On the other hand, I would turn fifty in August 2010, and I thought it might be fun to try Boston again, when I was at the low end of my age group. I was valuing the companionship of Janice's club runners and the idea of going as part of a group was appealing. Long runs were important for networking, and they were also giving me a foundation of some quality. I appreciated the benefits that came with group training, especially as our runs pushed out beyond two hours. I wasn't sure what kind of time I was still capable of, but it seemed worth finding out. I was still able to go under one hour thirty minutes for a half marathon, and I figured with some effort I could do better.

There seemed to be a fit in Janice's program, and I was keen to put her ideas to the test. On the other hand, my expectations for Boston had to be realistic. It would be my first marathon attempt in my fifties. And it had been more than seven years since the not entirely satisfying London Marathon in 2003. However, my dissatisfaction with that race had long since passed, and I felt ready to try again.

I set my sights on the 2010 Victoria Marathon, which would take place on October 10. Victoria had already been a successful venue for me, and I took the date 10-10-10 to be a further positive omen. It was bound to be a compelling race. As a first step, I ran the Calgary Marathon in May with a friend and former work colleague at Shell. Glen was developing into a capable runner, and he had set his sights on reaching a Boston Qualifier—a BQ—in what would be his first marathon. For me, the idea was to put a BQ in the bank and help pace Glen to our qualifying standard, which at the time was 3:35.

Our race started well, and our target pace was comfortable for me. I encouraged Glen as the morning went on. Sadly, he started having trouble with leg cramps around 30k. He eventually released me to finish on my own, about seven kilometres from the finish. I felt bad for him and would have stayed with him to the end. Instead, I was able to enjoy the uncommon experience of finishing a marathon strong and fresh, speeding up rather than hanging on for dear life. I finished thirty seconds under our BQ target. Glen missed achieving his own BQ by five minutes.

I had every reason to expect a better time in Victoria four months later. My training through the spring and summer had gone well, so there was reason to be optimistic. Race day dawned cool, breezy, and overcast. There was no hint of the rain or gale force winds that had been feared. While I would not say I felt bad in the early going, I started the morning with a sour stomach. A room service pizza is perhaps a bad choice at any time, but even more so as a pre-race meal. As a result, my first few kilometres were dodgy. My goal pace felt like more work than it should have. I didn't panic. By 5k I started feeling better, and at 10k I was back on target.

It was at this point that I started to realize how essential it had been to put a proper race plan together. I mentally thanked Janice. I had made some last-minute tweaks to the race plan we had agreed on, which would allow me to continuously remind myself of two things. First was the need to focus on form, which we did through a series of drills with the acronym SELF TALK. It was Smooth–Easy–Light–Fast as cues, and Tall–Arms–Lean–Knees for key elements of our running posture. I thought about four of my running heroes to give myself a mental picture: Seb Coe–Bill Rodgers–Haile Gebrselassie–Steve Prefontaine.

The second thing I tried to do was address the neck and shoulder pain on my left side, which had recently started to bother me in long training runs. At the time, I had no reason to think this pain was anything other than a result of fatigue or maybe poor posture, since it got worse in the later stages of long runs. Looking back now, I wonder if this pain may have been the earliest sign of the circulatory problem that eventually landed me in the stroke unit.

At the time, though, I had no idea what was causing the pain. My physiotherapist had given me a series of neck and shoulder exercises that we hoped would counteract the onset of fatigue, on the premise that that was the likely cause of the pain. I had been doing the exercises at home, even though they yielded little improvement in my condition. I came up with the idea of doing a couple of the exercises during the race. I added this to my plan. I would do a set of shoulder hunches and cross-over touches every five kilometres starting at the 5k mark. And I would alternate these with the form drills, every five kilometres starting at 8k.

Alternating my exercises worked like a charm. I was amazed at how soon the kilometre markers came up. It became like a small reward program in the middle of the race. I reached the halfway point comfortably in just under 1:33, then the turnaround point in the Uplands neighbourhood, and then the 28k mark, feeling physically strong.

More importantly, and unusually for this point in a marathon, I was mentally positive. On a whim, I started to wave and smile at the spectators. This was a bit out of character for me, but good for my morale. I remembered one of my teammates telling me that he swore by this tactic, particularly if he got a return wave from a pretty girl. That thought further lightened my spirit. Then, I was pleasantly surprised to see Janice and several of my teammates at the 32k mark. Their cheers were better fuel than the energy gel I had forced down minutes earlier.

I checked my pace. I had lost some time against my target between 28 and 35 kilometres, but only a minute or two. The small hills that had seemed like nothing on the way out had mysteriously grown in size on the way back. The wind, now in my face, was also a minor irritant. I told myself that none of that mattered because I was still feeling good. And I had evidence that this was true, since I seemed to be doing better than many runners around me. It was a rare marathon where I was able to pick people off in the late stages, but it was happening today.

Watch your form and relax, I told myself. SELF TALK! Remember Coe–Rodgers–Haile–Prefontaine!

The last part of my race plan included mental exercises, in which Janice wanted us to meditate about someone who had inspired us, then dedicate a couple of kilometres to someone important in our lives, and finally impersonate a favourite runner. The idea was to divert our minds away from any negative or self-defeating thoughts. Instead, we were to think about people that had been positive influences in our lives. Janice was my inspiration, given how much I appreciated her recent help in getting me to this point.

I had an unexpected result when I turned my mind to my father in the dedication phase. I chose Dad because he had passed away almost a year to the day of the race. As soon as I began to think about what he meant to me, and how much I owed him, I lost control. Tears streamed down my cheeks. There were no negative thoughts about Dad's personal failings, no despair over how he had died, no regrets about what might have been. Instead, I was overcome by warm feelings for my father. I saw how Dad had helped me to become the person I was. He had shown me that I should forge my own path and I knew, because I had done just that, that running had become my salvation and my refuge from the same fate he had suffered. I had taken full advantage of his example. Indeed, I was here because he had shown me it was okay to be my own person. My running in this race today was living proof of it.

Janice had asked me in our race planning session to consider whether this might be a bit too much to handle at the 35k mark of a marathon. It turned out she was right. I had never experienced such a swell of emotion in a race, but maybe it should not have been a surprise. I had been on the road for more than two hours, and the cumulative effect of the fatigue and Dad's loss was too overwhelming at that moment. I composed myself by saying a little goodbye to him, and by promising him that I would do my dedication later.

Meanwhile, the usually grim mid-thirties kilometres were sliding by with little noticeable loss of pace. Awesome! I had been looking forward to the impersonation phase for the whole race. My subject was Steve Prefontaine—forever known as Pre—the tenacious US distance runner, whose gutsy performance in the Munich 5000-metre Olympic final I could play on demand in my head, in grainy black and white footage, complete with play-by-play commentary. I combined thoughts of his aggressive running style with my form drill cues. I repeated, over and over again, like an impromptu mantra: Pre-Smooth, Pre-Easy, Pre-Light, and best of all, Pre-Fast. All the while I was passing other runners.

I carried my positive attitude all the way to the 41k mark.

Just over one kilometre to go! This was the point at which Janice had urged us to feel the pull of the finish line. I gave it all I had left, which was more than I had expected. I was thrilled to watch the 100-metre signs tick down. 700–600–500–. There was no feeling of strain. I was floating. 400–300–. I looked up for the finish banner. 200–100–. Just then, I *was* Pre, cruising effortlessly down the final straight.

I finished in 3:09, just under my optimistic goal time. Yes, it was well off my PB, set eighteen years earlier, but it was a solid performance. Better than solid. It was inspirational. Exhilarating. Here was by far the most consistent marathon I had ever run, and second only to Boston in 2001 as the most satisfying.

I learned that day that having a game plan, staying with it, and adapting it on the fly could help me surmount obstacles I had experienced time and again. I said a quiet thank you to Janice for teaching an old—well, aging—dog some new tricks. I thanked Dad properly in a moment of contemplation and prayer, later at my hotel. I also thought about my teammates, several of whom were running in the Chicago Marathon this same day. Only later would I learn what a tough day they'd had, fighting terrible weather conditions. For them, it was the kind of day when finishing was a major accomplishment.

My own experience on 10-10-10 was a revelation. I had made a huge step on the learning curve, which went well beyond the numbers. What I had done was remarkable. I had put *all* the pieces together and produced a result that I could be proud of.

My key personality traits had not changed: curiosity, diligence, humility. But on that day, I had moved beyond the physical act of running. I had added mental tactics that were as or more important. How could this have taken so long, and why had I been so unaware of the importance of these tools? It occurred to me that perhaps it was humility that mattered most. It had taken me many years to assemble all the pieces, and Janice had opened my eyes to the possibilities. Even if the marathon was still not my favourite race, the lessons learned could readily be applied to other races.

A few hours after the race, I eased my sore body into my seat for the short return flight to Calgary. I could begin to turn my mind toward the Boston Marathon in 2011. But first, I would savour this result. I felt immense satisfaction for what I had achieved, and pride for my teammates. On that day, we were all champions.

Tempting Fate

FOLLOWING MY SUCCESS IN VICTORIA, I was keen to put Janice's techniques to the test again soon. Boston was the goal in April 2011, but my teammates were full of ideas for other races. One race they mentioned in glowing terms was the "First Half" Half Marathon in Vancouver. I felt myself getting caught up in the excitement for this event. Because it is held in mid-February, it can be a good intermediate goal race for winter-weary Calgary runners. I secured a late entry through a lottery. Having this race in front of us was just the motivating factor my teammates and I needed to get through several long, frigid Sunday runs in December and January.

We had fun in Vancouver the day before the race. I was amused to learn that my lottery entry entitled me to bib number 3—a number usually reserved for elite athletes. I took this as an invitation, even though it meant I had to spend my warm-up deflecting glances from other runners who were clearly asking themselves who this speedster was. I put on my best "Don't worry, I'm not fast!" face.

In fact, the race did go well. While I didn't compete for top honours, I did hit all my splits and run a steady pace. The course, which was nostalgically marked in miles rather than kilometres, took us around scenic Stanley Park. It was a beautiful morning, the opposite of what I imagined we would have faced for our Sunday run had we been back in Calgary. I finished strong, in just under 1:26. It was a respectable result, an age group PB, and a confirmation of my fitness over what had been a bleak winter. As in Victoria four months earlier, I felt that I ran the whole race within my capabilities.

The First Half was one of the few races I knew of that published age-graded results, putting us older athletes on the same footing as the open competitors. I was elated to learn that I had run a time equivalent—almost to the second—to my all-time PB, by then almost twenty years in the past. Here was a tangible indicator of what I hoped were good things to come. But even that was not the best part of my day. Rather, it was meeting up with my teammates at the finish. All of us were delighted with our results. Adrenaline Rush was well represented at the award ceremony—so well that the announcer asked if we had chartered a plane from Calgary.

I hoped to use the First Half race as a solid foundation for the main event in Boston. As for Boston itself, I had no aspirations of getting close to the 2:58 that I had run when I was forty, even on an age-graded basis, because that day had been sublime. Perfect. Indeed, I was hesitant to go back to Boston. I was worried that this experience wouldn't match up to my first one. A small voice in my head asked if I was tempting fate.

Physically, things were mostly positive, but I had a few worries. There was that nagging pain in my left shoulder and neck, which had persisted throughout the winter. It had been joined since the previous autumn by a sharp, stabbing pain in the ball of my right foot, a pain that only bothered me on the downhills. Boston does have a lot of those. Knowing this, I decided to run the mileage, but not the hills, for the last two months of my training. Would this gamble pay off?

With considerable caution I made it through the subsequent

weeks of training, only to have a nasty tumble over a loose Great Dane who ran across the Bow River pathway right in front of me during our last interval session in early April. That fall aggravated the pain I had already been having in my left shoulder. I thought I had pulled a muscle, to add to whatever else had been giving me grief in that area.

Looking back on that incident, I can only wonder to what extent it exacerbated my later problems with an arterial blockage. Could I have damaged, or maybe further damaged, the artery when I went headfirst over that dog? It was certainly possible. It seems like more than a coincidence that I had such pain in the same area that would later debilitate me. Again, no one will ever be able to confirm whether my fall would have caused the later issues.

Despite this late setback, I made it through my taper and my race day preparations. The weather looked like it would cooperate—cool temperatures, partly cloudy and a slight wind from the west. We had a huge contingent of runners from Calgary in Boston that year. It was great to spend a couple of days with Deb and my teammates in one of our favourite cities. Deb and I decided to stay at the Lenox Hotel on Boylston Street, so that we could be close to the finish line. We found out that Copley Square was a very busy place on marathon weekend. Getting into the spirit of things, Deb ran in the BAA 5k race, one of the preliminaries before the big event. We even saw one of my heroes, Bill Rodgers, socializing with fans in the finish area as Deb finished her race.

What a sight the Adrenaline Rush group was in the athletes' village in Hopkinton, decked out in our club gear! My first Boston had been a solo experience. This time, it was more about celebrating with my new team. I felt that whatever was about to happen, I had already succeeded.

Since 2007, the BAA had abandoned the traditional noon start time for the marathon, in favour of earlier wave starts. This was a way to get more runners on the road. As a result, logistics on race morning were more complex than what I remembered in 2001. The start and the early miles were mostly about defensive running, in the close confines of 27,000 enthusiastic runners. At least I knew what to expect in the hectic crush of the early miles.

Around the five-mile mark, I spotted the distinctive singlets of a couple of my teammates, running side by side just up the road. I knew they were both hoping for a faster result than I was. I decided to keep them in sight a short distance ahead of me for a mile or two, then purposely let out a bit of line to widen the gap between us. I did not want to be tempted to overdo it. My early splits were on target, including 1:33 at the half. Had I eased off enough for the rigours still to come? There was no sign of trouble from my either my foot or my shoulder for the first half of the race. I was running the same pace as I had in Victoria, and, as I had done there, I used regular stretches to loosen my shoulder and drills to stay on form.

The day was turning out to be quite a bit warmer than expected, so I made sure to take in lots of water. In the Framingham flats, I noticed that my quads and knees were already sore. That was not an encouraging sign. I did some bum kicks as I ran, to try and loosen up. A few miles on, the women of Wellesley College were as loud and raucous as in 2001, but something seemed to be missing. I was not enjoying this race as much as I should. I told myself the problem was just nerves.

I felt some stings from my right foot around mile fourteen. I had no choice but to ignore the pain and carry on.

Stick to the race plan, I told myself. Use the mental tricks that worked so well in Victoria!

The Newton hills were tough—tougher than I remembered. The Boston that many runners feared was revealing its devious character today. Even as I watched my pace slowing, I told myself it was okay. After all, I had purposely avoided serious hill work just to get to the starting line. By the time I reached the top of Heartbreak Hill, I was beaten up, but happy to have it behind me. Today, there were to be no sightings of Dick and Rick Hoyt—Team Hoyt—although that special moment from the 2001 race still had the power to inspire me. From here, it was as simple as getting back on pace for the finish—one more ordinary forty-minute run would do it. After our heroic runs through the winter, wouldn't this be a breeze?

No.

It seemed I had nothing left. My confidence was eroding. I felt my field of vision narrowing. Even the crowds could not energize me. Instead, I found it all—the noise and the closeness of the other runners—to be disorienting. I had trouble dealing with the chaos on the racecourse, especially around the water stations. At one point, I was nearly tripped up by a runner who carelessly careened across the road directly in front of me. I had flashbacks of my encounter with that dog a couple of weeks earlier. As a race veteran, I should have been able to shake this incident off. Instead, it had the opposite effect. There were so many more runners around me than there had been ten years earlier. My race plan, which had so carefully laid out my nutrition and hydration intake, was all but forgotten. I let myself get rattled by the many distractions. I had lost my determination, my drive, and I couldn't get it back. Or maybe I just didn't care. I only wanted to see the finish line.

As I retreated into survival mode through the last few miles, my walk breaks became more frequent and longer. I thought about shutting off my watch. With a lot of bargaining—run to the next mile marker, run to the next water station, start running at the next corner—I somehow got to Hereford, made the final left turn, and jogged the long finish straight on Boylston. I had to acknowledge that the course had won on this day. I finished in 3:20.

Confidence is a fragile and elusive thing. It is hard to gain and harder to hold onto. Yet, it is a key ingredient for a successful race.

Like so many before me, I learned that running Boston could be a sobering experience. My 2011 result was twenty minutes slower and infinitely more difficult than my race ten years earlier. I could not reconcile how different these races felt. Maybe I had been so strong in the 2001 race that I just never noticed the many obstacles. I was reminded that it is important to have contingency plans in case things don't go as you expect. If there was one positive takeaway in 2011, it was the great support of my Adrenaline Rush teammates.

* * *

I was on a high after the Victoria Marathon, and the First Half race in February left me feeling optimistic about my training over the winter. Before Boston, I thought if I were to have a shot at another sustained period of peak performance, this might be it. And yet, I left Boston with my confidence in tatters. Nearly forty years on from my start in the sport, it was time to ask myself some serious questions. Competitive running had been the longest presence—the longest relationship, I could say—that I had had in my life, other than with my family. There had been ebbs and flows over the years, but there was a loyalty to this relationship that was extraordinary. But what had I really learned? After so many years and so many miles, could I still define a path to future success? There was no question that this relationship should continue, but what was I getting out of it, and what did I still want from it? What was I missing?

I thought about the things that had brought me the most satisfaction as a runner. I reminded myself that it often had little to do with the numbers. I had consistently gotten more fulfillment from the process of exploration, from the quest to define my own potential. I had never been a star, meaning that I was able to relish my anonymity while training or racing. Running was uncomplicated, I was part of it, and it brought me its own rewards. It seemed that whatever my way forward in the sport, I should make sure that it let me continue to capture these benefits.

I was proud of my historical success. I could rightly claim this success as my own, because for many years my approach to training was totally self-taught. For long periods, I relied on my wits to train and prepare for races. I was a dedicated student of the sport. I had figured out the elements that needed to be in my training program, and most of the time I could trust that I got the balance of the elements right. Sometimes I did miss one element or another, and no doubt that omission was reflected in my race results, but my ad hoc approach never led me too far astray. I was fully invested in my own success. I was not content to just look back, though. I knew that I still wanted to test my own limits and accomplish more in the sport.

For years, I had insisted on doing many long runs alone, knowing that on race day it would come down to how well I performed on my own. But paradoxically, although running is the essence of an individual sport, I realized how much value I had gained from being part of a team. In high school, I first experienced the intensity of feeling that came from being part of something bigger than myself. Years later, being part of an active local club, and participating on memorable mountain relay teams had allowed me to recapture those feelings, even if fleetingly. And then, the feeling of satisfaction that came from working with my friends to tackle a gruelling interval workout, or to complete an epic long run when Calgary's winter weather was doing its utmost to upset our plans. These too were moments to be proud of, forged through shared adversity and fuelled by camaraderie. I knew I wanted that to continue.

I thought about the talented coaches who had guided me at different points in my running life: Mr. James, Ray and Gord, Mahedi, and most recently Janice. The events of the last few months had reminded me how many elements need to come together for success. It was easy to be overwhelmed, as had just happened to me in Boston. It was invaluable to have someone help set the foundation, organize the building, offer constructive advice, and adjust the program along the way to keep me on target for execution. My relationships with helpers and mentors were special, and built on mutual trust. My coaches were very different people from one another, each with their own approaches, but they all had one thing in common—an unswerving dedication to the task of making each of us, making me, a better runner.

For my part, I put great stock in being accountable for delivering my best every day. I call my attitude being coachable. That was not always easy, particularly for true amateur athletes like me, as we juggled running with the other elements of our lives. However, coachability is rooted in humility, something that I do understand. With Adrenaline Rush, I had been doubly lucky. I had a great coach in Janice, who understood how to get the best out of her athletes. And I had fallen in with a supportive group of teammates that were committed to helping each other succeed. I wanted to do my best for them, as much as for myself.

There was one other thing. Maybe because I had started running in the days before technology dramatically changed the sport, I tended not to stress too much about tracking or recording my statistics. There were weeks, even years, when I didn't worry excessively about distance and pace. Admittedly, that was getting harder to do with a GPS watch on every runner's wrist, including mine most of the time. Rather than adding to the experience it was starting to feel like I was losing something. I reminded myself that unless I was building up to a goal race, not every workout needed to be recorded. The pace for each kilometre I ran was irrelevant. When it was important to sweat the details, I did. And I still could.

But I couldn't deny that a little voice was already telling me that I might be happier with fewer big race buildups. Or maybe I just needed some different running experiences. Hadn't I already achieved quite a lot? Why not just simplify things, get out and enjoy running for its own sake? In doing so, maybe I could recapture a little lost freedom.

* * *

I regrouped after Boston and recommitted to Janice's program. With her help, I began to approach racing in a different, more systematic way. My hope was that the inevitable slow decline in my performances could be made up for by a smarter, more complete approach to racing. There was still much more for me to learn. By incorporating the necessary elements into my training, I felt I was giving myself the best chance for success.

Janice and I had developed a productive partnership. Because she respected that I had decades of running experience, she tended not to tell me what to do. Rather, with her coach's sense of how to motivate her athletes, she led me to see that race preparation was a continuous process, comprising many small steps. What she may not have fully appreciated was how much I welcomed direction, especially if it would help make me a better, more complete runner. As a task-oriented person, I worked better when I had a job to do. I had let myself get into race situations in which I was merely reacting, rather than actively anticipating events. Instead, I could rely on my race plan as a way of keeping myself on target. It was necessary to be flexible and adjust the plan on the go, as I had done in Victoria in 2010. Sure, I had slipped up in Boston six months later, but that was no big deal. This was a process and there would be setbacks.

Over the subsequent period, my whole approach to running, as well as my philosophy of life, started to come into sharper focus. It was only the start though, because I could not have fully verbalized what process was underway to bring about these changes. It would take the events of 2017 to fully crystallize the ideas that I can now see clearly in the rear-view mirror.

* * *

The soul-searching I did after Boston in the spring and summer of 2011 was born out of an attempt to reap more benefits from my athletics training. I hoped to incorporate new ideas I'd picked up from Janice into my existing regimen. Unbeknownst to me at the time, I would need this reset, as I was about to enter one of the most difficult periods of my personal and professional life. Competitive running was only one thread in a patchwork of challenges that were to intersect in rather chaotic fashion over the subsequent years.

For some time, I had managed to find a balance, barely, between my increasingly busy work schedule and a home life that was only slightly more predictable. Deb had embarked on a new career as a flight dispatcher with a major airline. This was another of her impressive career shifts. She was doing important and satisfying work, and while she was rightly proud of her achievements, her schedule of twelve-hour shifts was daunting. Thankfully, our sons were both on their own and becoming well-established in their careers. They did not need our constant attention any longer. We could not have been prouder of them.

Running after work and on weekends had become the norm for me, as I was finding it nearly impossible to tear myself away the office during the day. I had to be content with the fond memories of my lunchtime runs out of the downtown Y. At Purvin & Gertz, my partners and I had earned much success, but we were a small firm in an industry where uncertain times were seemingly never far off in the future. For this reason, we gave serious consideration to an acquisition offer that was made by a large energy insight firm shortly after the 2011 Boston Marathon. By then, I had progressed to the position of director, so besides my involvement in ongoing strategic and operational issues I found myself fully immersed in our review of the proposed deal. It was a hectic year.

We accepted the offer late in 2011 and began integrating ourselves into the multinational firm that had acquired us. There were many hurdles throughout this process. Culturally, our firms could not have been more different. I was inundated by conflicting demands, all of which seemed to find their way to my desk. I felt my loyalty was with the local staff I had previously managed. This period was destined to become the most arduous of my professional life, and I let the worst aspects of this transition spill over into my family life. I was wrong to let my work troubles affect my relationship with Deb and the boys, but I had let this happen. I was miserable, and I know for much of the time I was not fit to live with. I needed to find a way out of this situation. I began looking for other opportunities.

In contrast to the professional issues that I was dealing with, and not always successfully, I continued to find solace in running. Just as at previous challenging times, running became the one thing that kept me grounded during this period. I clung to the structure of regular workouts through the weeks of the Adrenaline Rush race buildup, as that was one place that I felt truly comfortable. Tuesdays were reserved for strength sessions, usually hills or strides, with a focus on good running posture. Thursday evenings were set aside for interval training. Almost as soon as we had finished a session in Prince's Island Park or at the Olympic Oval, I began to look forward to the next one. Sunday long runs were a fixture. For me, a Sunday run was a small luxury that I treated myself to, an opportunity to get lost in conversation with my teammates as we cruised along the river pathways. Our runs sometimes stretched to three hours or more. To be consistent with my renewed commitment to a more flexible approach on other days, I ran when I could and managed to keep my fledgling streak going.

* * *

In 2012, searching for a novel running experience, I decided it would be fun to have a rematch with my sixteen-year-old self and run the Around the Bay Race again. My objective was simple: to beat my time from thirty-five years earlier. In the interim, the race had been standardized to the 30k distance. It was long, but not marathon long. The race had also morphed from a local curiosity, of interest only to several hundred scraggly diehards, into a major event on the Ontario race calendar. My training base was solid enough that I decided to give it a try.

I managed to eke out a small victory in the virtual head-to-head match up, running 2:15 but finishing well down in the age group results. As I plodded through the latter stages of the race, I felt myself being transported back to that cold day in March so many years earlier. I was thankful for the advances in technology since 1977, even if the better fabrics and electronics seemed to be making little difference to my performance. In what might have been an experimental test of the longevity of muscle memory, my exhausted legs seemed to relive every rolling hill on North Shore Boulevard. I crested the final hill on Spring Garden Road, leaving only three kilometres to reach the downtown finish inside the Copps Coliseum. I laughed as I ran by a costumed Grim Reaper who was standing next to the cemetery gate on York Boulevard and yelling at us to "D-I-E a little out there!" I let this amusing encounter be the beginning of my celebration of this day, this opportunity, this adventure. I was overcome by the gamut of emotions. Where had all the time gone?

Although I had long since accepted that marathons were not my strong suit, the lure of running another one would occasionally call out to me in a moment of weakness. More than once I had sworn "no more marathons," usually right after finishing one and sometimes for years thereafter. True to form, then, I found that my less than satisfying race in Boston in 2011 had dampened my enthusiasm for the marathon for a while. Sometimes, though, the motivation comes from a different place than you expect.

Our son, Dan, was developing into a fine runner in his own right. He had started running with a club in Montreal that was affiliated with the McGill University cross-country and track teams. That led to a call for him to try out for the varsity team. He made the cut, and promptly began to put together an impressive string of personal bests.

Deb and I recalled the chubby kid who had shown little initial promise as a runner. Years earlier, while we were living in the UK, Dan had trudged through a middle school cross-country season, being humoured by his classmates and teachers. What was notable about that experience was how it revealed his true character. He internalized a commitment to improve for the next year. He took the coach's advice to run for thirty days and tripled it. He ran every day over the summer, most of the time with Deb. By summer's end they were both fit and he was more than ready for the start of the new season. His classmates barely recognized him.

That determined kid was apparently still at it. Our first true head-to-head race, and another new experience for me, was the Stampede 5k Road Race in 2012. I thought leading from the front would be my best tactic and my only hope. I spent three kilometres looking over my shoulder and running for my life. It was no surprise when Dan flew by me as we approached the 4k mark. It was with a combination of parental pride and utter despair that I realized I had no response to his surge. He told me later he had pressed the issue as he went by me, knowing that I would put up some resistance. I wish, I said to myself.

In rapid succession, Dan ran a couple of races that put to rest for good any debate about where things stood in the family running standings. First, he and I signed up for the Bay Race early in the 2014 season. This was a real lesson in humility for me, as I laboured from start to finish, while Dan crushed his race, running 1:57. My sister Carolyn and her daughter were with Deb at the finish to share this experience with us. Later in the year, he ran his first marathon in Montreal. Once again, he nailed it. His disciplined approach to the race meant that he ran a perfectly even pace. Besides being exceedingly rare, his performance was totally opposite to my own first marathon in Toronto—that dreadful effort from thirty-two years earlier. Dan held his pace for the entire race, and finished tenth overall, in 2:51. In his first marathon, his result was better by almost a minute than my PB, which had taken me *five* tries to reach.

It wasn't a surprise, then, when Dan set his sights on running Boston in 2016. I'm not sure exactly where the idea of my going to Boston with him originated. Regardless, it was a brilliant idea. I had no valid reason to say no, so I agreed. There would be the small obstacle of running a qualifying race first. I tried not to dwell on that, or the ribbing that my teammates would dish out when I shared the news that I was once again going to tackle the marathon. I could hear them already: "You said you'd never run another marathon!"

I chose the 2015 Vancouver Marathon as my Boston qualifier. It was a safe choice for a spring race and popular with Calgary runners. Getting ready was an odd combination of being in decent physical shape, but not being all that confident. My last data point had been the humbling 2014 Bay Race. Again, I was experiencing self-doubt. And once again, it was the encouragement of my teammates that helped me find the fortitude to sign up for the race. Allison and Ken were my constant companions on long runs through the winter and early spring. Allison was just beginning to find her groove as a marathoner. She would also be racing in Vancouver, and she would soon be achieving world-class age group times. Ken was well on his way towards his goal of running sixty marathons before his sixtieth birthday. I could not have asked for two better training partners in the weeks leading up to the race.

Race day dawned cool and bright. I felt good for the first ten kilometres, where the course elevation dropped steadily, mimicking Boston's profile. I tried to coast to save energy, running in what Janice liked to call *tourist mode*. I was on pace, if maybe a bit fast. A medium-sized hill that began at the 10k mark was an early test. I noticed the effort, but it was manageable. By the 16k mark, I was ready to push things. Janice and I had agreed on a creative race plan that included a series of four 3k pickups, each followed by a 1k recovery. Here was another example of her ingenuity. She had found a way to get the best out of me, by giving me small tasks in the middle of the race. I used the 3k sections to push the pace and pass some people. The recovery sections became something to look forward to, like small rewards for my effort. I steadily moved up through the field and was buoyed by the feeling of being in control as I did so.

I passed through the half in 1:36, meaning that I was on target to run about 3:15. I did my best to enjoy the scenic course. In what might have been another early warning of the problems I would experience a couple of years later, I had a strange feeling of disorientation—mild vertigo—for about half a kilometre at the 24k mark. It passed quickly. (I never thought about it again until I set out to write this narrative.)

Coming off the Burrard Bridge at 30k, I regrouped for one more test—the final kilometres along the Stanley Park Seawall. I thought about Allison, running up the road somewhere ahead of me. Her running technique is exceptional, and I tried to use that mental picture to keep myself on form. By 38k, my quads began to seize up. I didn't panic. I knew that I could still finish well if I managed my effort over the last few kilometres. I might miss my optimistic goal time, but so be it—this was about qualifying for Boston. Soon enough, I caught sight of the finish banner—as welcome as ever—and I crossed the line in 3:18. Allison was already relaxing in the finish area, having finished seven minutes earlier.

Overall, I was happy with my performance, and I felt like it did me good to commit to the race. I had beaten my BQ standard by a very comfortable twenty-two minutes, while Dan had beaten his own by a mere fifteen minutes. I made sure to point this out to him in a good-natured way. We both looked forward to meeting up in Boston the following April.

The Power of Running

RUNNING BECAME EVEN MORE of a sanctuary for me in 2015. I continued to pursue various career opportunities as they came up, since my interest in the status quo had long since waned. As a result, I was short-listed for an appointment as a Board Member at Canada's National Energy Board, or NEB. This was a position I knew I would be a strong candidate for, based on my long stint of nearly two decades as an independent energy consultant.

I was honoured when I received word that summer that I was a successful candidate for the NEB role. I began to look forward to the next phase of my career serving the Canadian public. However, the transition was not destined to be a smooth one. For some time, the strong reputation of the agency had been under attack by various special interest groups. Furthermore, in my opinion, an overly zealous new federal government had begun to undermine the work of the agency. I saw this as reckless and inappropriate.

It was a difficult time to join the NEB. Initially, I relied on my great confidante, solo running, to help me make sense of a complex situation. I knew that my mind would inevitably take its own course while I ran. My fresh musings about the meaning and purpose of life found a sympathetic ear in the companion who steadfastly accompanied me on the road, a trusted advisor who always had my best interests at heart.

Here was a case where I found I could apply lessons learned over a lifetime in amateur sports to the professional realm—trust in myself, work hard, stay modest. I was soon vindicated in my belief that I could contribute meaningfully to the agency's important work of regulating Canada's energy systems. I went out of my way to share the benefits of my experience with NEB staff, most of whom appreciated my efforts. Despite a lot of external noise and the resulting stress that this created, my time at the agency would ultimately prove to be satisfying.

* * *

My qualifying time for the 2016 Boston Marathon was respectable. Given my trying work situation, I found myself with plenty of impetus, but perhaps less time than I would have liked, to log the necessary training hours. Even so, five weeks before the race, I developed Achilles tendonitis. This had become a recurrent problem, which I instinctively knew was due to two factors. The first was overtraining on aging legs. The second was my rather lax approach to strength training as a supplement to my running. Whatever the reasons, when it returned in March 2016, the tendonitis was serious enough to sabotage my marathon training. By early April, I was making a frustratingly slow recovery, and I wasn't sure I would be able to run. I faced a growing dilemma. If I could get the injury sorted out in time, it would mean tackling the demanding Boston course on almost no training.

Meanwhile, Dan continued to thrive as a distance runner. He had trained with conviction, through the worst of a Montreal winter. He aspired to run an exceptional time in Boston—about 2:40, he had declared—in what would be only his second marathon. This was an audacious, even brash, prediction, but he was on track to do it. His training had gone extremely well, and he was ready.

Of course, because this would be my third Boston, I thought I knew what to expect. In truth, I was not overly keen to run the race again. I had entered mainly to be part of Dan's experience. Deb was perhaps the most excited, as she would see us both run this historic race. As we had done in 2011, we booked a room at the Lenox Hotel, a few steps from the finish line. For Deb and me this race was really about Dan. I was content to play a supporting role.

On April 17, the day before the race, with my Achilles tendon feeling almost normal, I made the decision to go ahead with it. Dan and I took one last jog around the Common. As had become our custom, we enjoyed an Italian meal in Boston's North End and went to bed early.

Race day Monday was warm, sunny, and breezy. I had been lucky over the years when it came to marathon day weather, and today was shaping up to be decent. Our nerves were calm on the lengthy bus ride to the start in Hopkinton. We didn't talk much. Each of us was preoccupied with our own thoughts. In the five years since I had last run the race, the field size had swelled even more, so for this 120th edition there would be something like 30,000 runners going through the athletes' village. Dan and I were in different start waves. His faster qualifying time meant that he would start thirty minutes ahead of me.

We said a slightly awkward goodbye and wished each other luck. Thinking about the obstacles that were ahead, and about how my last Boston experience had foundered after I lost focus on my race plan, I tried to offer Dan a few last words of fatherly advice. I told him to trust his training and respect the course. He was not hearing much of anything at that point. Mostly, I was hoping that he would not let his adrenaline push him too fast in the early going, although I kept that thought to myself.

I had only minimal expectations for myself. Finishing would be enough today. Could I even run? The early downhill miles would be my first real test in weeks. I was feeling fine and thanks to steady doses of Tylenol, I had no Achilles pain. My improvised race plan, devised that morning, was to reach the top of Heartbreak Hill at mile twenty-one without walking, and then jog-walk to the finish. By chance, I met a runner from my 1988 Jasper–Banff Relay team as we made the slow walk to the starting corrals. I had not seen Kim for years. He had since retired. Like me, he had dealt with some injuries on his journey to Boston, so we commiserated a little and wished each other well. Positive thoughts of that memorable race could only help me today.

I started very conservatively and made it to the halfway mark in 1:44. I was still relatively comfortable, even though my pace was already slowing. I did my best to absorb some energy from the Wellesley scream tunnel. I could really use some help from the enthusiastic young women this time around, given my worries about the challenges yet to come. My hamstrings and quads seemed not to get the message, though. They were tightening up badly, victims of my poor fitness and the fiendish topography of Boston. The warm, dry conditions were having a dehydrating effect, so I made a point of overcompensating by drinking a lot of water. I hoped Dan was doing the same, miles up the road.

By mile seventeen, my lack of fitness got the better of me. Yes, this had happened earlier than I'd hoped, but it was not a surprise. I felt no guilt as I took full advantage of walk breaks on the Newton hills. With more than a little relief I reached the top of Heartbreak. I pulled off the road and stretched out my tight muscles for a minute before resuming the struggle. From there, it was the slow slog to the finish I had expected. Unlike in 2011, the crowds and the chaos around me didn't disrupt my race plan. This time, I was waging a private battle. My walk breaks became longer and more frequent, and I watched the minutes ticking by. I made a bargain with myself that I would not let myself go over four hours. At a few points even that seemed up for debate.

Eventually, finally, I reached the now-familiar turns, right on Hereford, left on Boylston. What a welcome sight! I gave myself full credit for managing to get through this. With the finish now only minutes away, I soaked up the celebratory atmosphere of what I knew would be my last Boston Marathon finish. In the moment, I felt pure joy and pride, for myself and my son. The only motivation I had needed to get here was the thought of Dan finishing the race ahead of me. That picture, the one with us and our medals, was already clear in my mind—

I finished in 3:51, a slow time for me but a finish all the same. The second half of the race had been a grim two-hour ordeal. Exhaustion, tinged with relief, weighed on me in the long finish chute. My Achilles had held up surprisingly well. On seized post-marathon legs, I hobbled back to the hotel as fast as I could. The enhanced security around the finish line since the appalling terrorist attack on the marathon in 2013 meant that my short walk to the hotel seemed to take forever. Hurry!

As soon as Deb answered the door, it was obvious something was wrong.

"Where's Dan?" I asked. He should have been there already.

She had just received a call from a nearby hospital. In fact, she already suspected there was a problem, since she had been monitoring Dan's progress online, and had not seen him at the finish when she expected. He was okay, the nurse said—thank God! —but he had collapsed on the course. Dan came on the phone and said that he remembered weaving around the road at twenty-three miles, then waking up in a medical tent. An ambulance was there to take him to the hospital. They would release him only when he was rehydrated, and they would deliver him directly to our hotel. We would have to wait.

We were in shock. This was not how things were supposed to turn out. Wasn't he the sure bet? Wasn't I the questionable one to finish? When Dan arrived back at the room in hospital scrubs a little while later, there were tears in the room. He looked and felt fine. He told us that he had started to feel bad early in the race. He thought he was losing time, so he kept pushing himself harder, not wanting to disappoint his teammates. He passed countless runners on the hills, and with three miles to go he told himself to just put up with another twenty minutes of pain. He never made it.

The mood for the rest of our trip was subdued. We put on brave faces. I had already stashed my medal away and vowed never to look at it. Dan was sombre. Deb was heartbroken. As we talked, we realized that Dan had run a daring and courageous race. Although his youth and inexperience had cost him a finish, he had proven that he belonged in Boston. He had made us extremely proud, just as he had been doing his whole life. But how would he handle this setback?

By the next day, he had talked to his coach and teammates, and he was coming to terms with the situation. Deb and I were already looking on the bright side. After all, this was one race. Dan was healthy, and that was all that mattered. He would be smarter and stronger the next time. We were quite sure there would be another Boston in his future. We even declared our intention to be there, to cheer him across the finish line.

* * *

My mind was teeming in the aftermath of the 2016 Boston Marathon. What should I do next? Could I even continue to race, with an Achilles tendon condition that had started to flare up quite regularly? And what about Daniel? I felt partly responsible for his race day misfortune. Running wasn't my only source of anxiety. I had experienced many twists of fate in the preceding few years, both positive and negative. Fortunately, by the summer, my work situation had improved. I had settled into the stringent processes of the regulatory world. It was meaningful and satisfying work, and I was good at it. I was proud of my contributions, and I made a point of ignoring the static that continued to swirl around the agency.

Our adventure in Boston led me to think about Dan's ascent through the ranks of competitive running, which by then seemed to be matched by my own decline. The 2016 race had been shaping up as a metaphor for the relative arcs of our lives. I imagine there are all sorts of philosophical overtones that could be applied to this story. The irony that I was hobbled by an Achilles tendon injury, like the hero of Greek mythology, invulnerable except for his heel, was not lost on me.

If I was looking for life lessons, it was worth remembering how this episode ended. After all, hadn't I persevered to the finish? There is dignity that comes from simply running the race. We participate, just as we live. We do not know what the result will be, and that is why we make the effort. For me, there had been no other option. I had experienced the full range of outcomes and emotions, from the euphoric result of my first Boston Marathon in 2001 to the satisfaction of a team effort in 2011 to the bittersweet turn of events in 2016, all on the same stretch of road between Main Street in Hopkinton and Boylston Street in Boston. Beyond that, I could count numerous highs, plenty of ordinary results, and my share of disappointments. In my life story, distance running had become the ideal proxy.

In the end, my decision on the way forward was unequivocal. There was no doubt that I needed to keep running and, barring injury, I hoped to continue competing. My marathoning days were behind me—this time I meant it—but it was with a renewed sense of purpose that I told Janice at the start of our fall session that I wanted to concentrate on shorter 5k and 10k races. There was no shortage of competition and more scope for racing strategy at these distances as compared to the marathon, which usually came down to hanging on as long as possible. It was appealing to think about trying different tactics.

This seemed to be a practical response and a reasonable way forward. Just thinking about shorter races rejuvenated my competitive spirit and provided another validation for what I had always felt about competing: I did not need to follow the pack. It was up to me to decide where to apply my talents. I approached 2017 with enthusiasm for new pursuits. In what might be the ultimate twist of fate, I never got a chance to put that commitment into action.

* * *

My late sister Carolyn was five years younger than me. I remember her as a cute, happy, and independent kid. In my favourite photograph of our family, that one from my first communion, she is just in front of me, a two-year-old in pigtails, with her bubbly personality on full display. As is clear from that picture, she was content to be part of the family. More than that, to be enveloped by us. I imagine given the full house we all lived in, that must have been a bit overwhelming for her at times. Still, she seemed to adapt well, even thrive, as younger siblings often do.

Carolyn was most like our grandmother, a person content to live in the moment, and to experience life passionately. I feel like I missed Carolyn's formative years while I was busy with my own pursuits during high school and university. I can rationalize that now by telling myself that things worked out such that I never really knew her well. After all, I had moved west before she was finished school. As our families grew up, I came to appreciate her love of life, her conviction to her ideals, and her devotion to her kids. That was despite the physical distance that was between us.

My fondest memories of Carolyn come from a period when she took up running. I don't think she was even in her teens. By then running was quite familiar in our house, so she may have wanted to emulate Paul and me. The reason she started running doesn't matter. She took to the sport and went on to assemble a daily streak that eventually stretched to ten years. Most of her runs were done as laps around Gage Park, where she often pushed herself to ten miles or more. She was running more than I was. Her willpower was astonishing. Carolyn had the toughness of Jerome Drayton.

The horrible period that led to her untimely passing started in early 2016, when she was diagnosed with a rare, aggressive sarcoma. How was this possible? The fear, the shock, the total helplessness that I'd felt after our sister Kathleen's strikingly similar diagnosis decades earlier were rekindled in an instant. In Carolyn's case, her disease was so rare that the doctors could not give her much of a read on her prognosis. It didn't take much medical expertise to see that her prospects were poor. The surgery and the radiation that they administered right away were feeble weapons against this enemy. What a cruel hand she had been dealt. And despite that, when I spoke to her, she was still the sweet, caring, soft-spoken, principled girl from our childhood.

Although no one would have said it out loud, we all determined to do our best to enjoy whatever time we had left with Carolyn. That would turn out to be only a couple of years. It was somehow fitting that for a brief period during her treatments, she felt well enough to run an 8k road race in Burlington. She later told me that was the one day she felt the most alive during the sad, hard days that she spent fighting cancer. The power of running, indeed.

Putting the Pieces Back Together

I GOT MY DISCHARGE from the hospital on July 28, 2017. A day earlier, I learned that the doctors had reached a consensus on my treatment plan. They decided the best way forward was to rely on medication to prevent any further strokes. Although stenting my vertebral artery was feasible, the procedure would be risky. Given the configuration of the arteries and the location of the blockage, the doctors told me a stent would have to be inserted from above. They didn't have to say much more. I thought about my compromised artery weaving its way through the vertebrae in my neck and up into my brain. Where would *above* even be, I wondered. At the same time, with no plan to repair the defect, I felt I was being handed a very uncertain future. It had barely been a week since my last TIA. Did we have enough evidence that medication alone would work?

There were a few final checks before I could leave the hospital. I welcomed the help of the health care experts who were there to ease my transition back to normal life. After seventeen days, I questioned what normal life was going to be, or if it was even possible. First, I had a mandatory lecture on managing my warfarin dosage. I learned about the foods and beverages I should avoid, and the details of the blood testing protocol I would have to follow while on the drug. I began to see why warfarin has a bad reputation.

I met again with the therapists whose job it was to make sure I could perform basic tasks. They watched me walk and climb stairs. They gave me a cognitive test. I let my engineer's brain take over, and I immediately messed it up. The puzzled look on the therapist's face said it all. I eventually recovered and finished the test with a flourish, much to her relief. She also explained the rules for driving after having a stroke. For now, I was grounded.

Another neurologist, Dr. Hill, whom I had not met before, spoke to us before my discharge. During our conversation, he ventured a hypothesis for my blocked artery that made a lot of sense. Given the configuration of my arteries, specifically the fact that I have only one vertebral artery to feed the basilar artery, he suggested that the blood flow in that artery had likely been higher than it would be for a person who had two arteries doing the same job. Then there was the junction between the subclavian and vertebral arteries—the design that I had described as flawed to Dr. Demchuk—which Dr. Hill felt could have further increased the stress at that point. Combined, these factors may have caused the damage to my artery, perhaps due to turbulent blood flow. This explanation sounded reasonable, and somehow it sat better with me than just chalking it all up to bad genes. At the end of the day, the cause was irrelevant, because it didn't change my situation or what we might do going forward.

It had seemed strange to find myself in the stroke unit, but it now seemed even stranger to be walking out with my small bag of belongings. Deb picked me up from the side door of the hospital, and as we made our way home, I felt that familiar roads had somehow changed over the last three weeks. I watched people driving and walking the streets on this warm summer day. Just then, the magnitude of the tectonic shift in my world became clear—I was watching my former life through the car window. A feeling of loss and detachment overwhelmed me.

The next few days were consumed with slowly getting back into my domestic routine. I appreciated having something real to occupy my mind. I knew Deb was happy to have me back in the house, and I was happy to be there. I called friends and relatives to let them know the latest news and my status. I continued the pleasant habit of an afternoon nap, for at least a while longer.

To ease my return home, my colleague Phil lent me an iPod with a couple of audiobooks. I listened to a murder mystery that was set in the Covent Garden area of London. The story took me back to our lived experience in the UK years earlier. Denmark Street, with its music shops, and the bustling Leicester Square Tube station—I had walked those same streets many times during our UK adventure. The audiobook was a welcome diversion.

* * *

I was home, and I was apparently still me. But there were many questions that we had left unasked, intentionally, until then. What were my true capabilities? What could I handle at work? What if I were to have more attacks?

Then there were the running questions. How would I react when this activity, one that had such a prominent role in my life, had been wrenched away from me? What would come after? These had moved from abstract hypotheticals to concrete questions. How any of us would feel—having had something that we consider to be a significant part of what defines us, abruptly taken away—says much about our worldview and our maturity as fully formed human beings. These were questions I was about to explore for the first time.

For the preceding four decades, I might have gone so far as to say that I could not continue to live without running in my life. My connection with the sport had been formed early in my life and had only grown stronger with time. I expected to be a competitive runner until my last days. For now, at least, that seemed beyond my grasp. I had no psychological mechanism to deal with this new reality.

I knew about the model that described the different stages of grief, and I recognized myself going through some of those stages. Several times, I had denied that I'd even had a stroke. I had reacted with unjustified anger when the doctors dared to order more tests. I remember bargaining with someone, I suppose that was God, that if he didn't take any more of my brain— "please, no more white spots on an MRI"—then I would try to be a better person when this was over. I understood that the final stage of grief is acceptance, but I wasn't sure where I was yet, in terms of accepting the reality of my new situation.

I did know that I was extraordinarily lucky, and for several reasons. First, although it was difficult to count the exact number of TIAs I had suffered until the doctors stabilized me—it was at least eight—I had reason to believe that I had not been permanently debilitated. Second, while the doctors had not felt it necessary to impose any strict limits on me, they had sent me home with the helpful advice that I not do anything stupid. Okay, so no rugby or skydiving. What that left me with was yet to be determined. As I would soon learn, my boundaries would be set by my own confidence, not by any rulebook.

Since there was nothing to do but find out, Deb and I began to explore my limitations. The first few days, we took tentative walks around the block. Then we set our sights on doing a lap around South Calgary Park, just across Fourteenth Street from our house, a distance of about one kilometre. It must have been tough for Deb to walk at my laboured pace. As slow as I was, I had to take frequent breaks to deal with the same unnerving feeling I had been experiencing since my last TIA two weeks earlier, of being pitched forward by a pair of invisible hands on my collar and waist. I would stop and sit on a bench or lean on a tree until the feeling passed. Despite my wobbles, we persevered and made our daily walks a priority.

* * *

August 6 was my fifty-seventh birthday. Janice had arranged a get-together for the running group at her spacious house on Lake Chaparral, south of Calgary. It was a Sunday and that meant the group would do a long run together. That day, a potluck brunch would follow for friends and family. Some brave souls would take a dip in the lake. I was excused from the run, even though everyone knew I would have been there with them under normal circumstances.

Deb and I joined the group after their run. I looked around at my friends and teammates as we walked into the back yard. They were as fit a group as I could find anywhere. Everyone was relaxed and talkative after their workout. I thought about all we had achieved together. I began to feel, for the first time, the full weight of my loss.

Nothing can ever be the same again, I thought. I felt myself tearing up.

The joy that came from being there and seeing everyone was mixed with immense sadness. I was with them, but from that point on I would be apart from them. They were the same. I was not. Many of my teammates had not seen me since we had run together in the Kananaskis relay in June, right before my hospital stay. I wondered what they were expecting to see, knowing that I had been in the stroke unit. As I chatted with each of them, I sensed over and over their genuine relief to see me looking fine, at least to outward appearances. I thought this might make me feel better too. Instead, all I noticed was the chasm that had opened between us.

No one knew it was my birthday, but Deb must have let the word get out. The whole group broke into a spontaneous and heartfelt rendition of *Happy Birthday.* I fought back the tears, yet again. Maybe some of my friends guessed, correctly, that I was getting my wish by just being there, nine days after my discharge. Then Janice presented me with my medal from the relay. I had almost forgotten the feelings of happiness and pride from that day, when we finished first in the Masters' 50+ category. It seemed so long ago. While I put on a brave face, I felt myself reaching a new low. This bit of shiny metal was a symbol of my loss. Anxiety deepened into panic, and I was relieved when we left soon after.

* * *

We continued our daily walks. Gradually we were able to add an extra block, then two. The streets of our neighbourhood, which are rather hilly, were a greater impediment at walking pace than I had ever noticed when running here. Deb was patient with me, more than I was with myself. I hoped that I hadn't already reached my limit.

As slow and frustrating as my physical progress was, I felt normal mentally. I was ready to return to the office and believed I was equal to the challenge, but there were many unknowns. I knew I would rather occupy my mind with practical matters than with self-defeating thoughts. For a couple of weeks, Deb was a sport—she dropped me off and picked me up. Then, feeling that I had imposed on her enough, I took the plunge and rode the bus, solo. Since I had been a bus rider for so many years growing up, this was not a burden. I imagined myself back on the Hamilton Street Railway and secretly enjoyed having ten minutes to myself, to read a couple of pages of a book or check my emails.

As for the work, I found I could do the job, but it was difficult to concentrate for extended periods. I also found that I was totally fatigued after even a few hours in the office. My fellow board members stepped up and showed themselves to be exemplary colleagues—they assumed my duties on the more pressing files and let me ease back into the work environment when and as I felt ready. I also appreciated the efforts of the NEB staff, who rearranged or deferred my other duties such as committee work.

* * *

Little mention had been made of running for a month. Then came the day I had been thinking about since July 10, the last day of my streak. It was August 27. Deb and I had both known this day was coming and suddenly it arrived. We knew it was time. It had been exactly a month since I was released from the hospital, five weeks since my last attack, and just two months since that memorable day at the relay with my teammates. It was still hard to believe what I had been through since then.

With more than a little trepidation, I pulled on my favourite North Face shorts and Adidas technical shirt. I laced up my Asics DS-Trainers and put on my Garmin GPS watch. Given how far we were about to run, none of that was really necessary. I could have done this run in my jeans and street shoes. To me, putting each of these things on was a symbolic act, more than an actual need.

I'M GOING FOR A RUN, I said to myself. The phrase, uttered thousands of times before, had never been so meaningful.

Deb was with me every step of the way. We managed a very slow jog around the block, once, a total distance of about five hundred metres. We walked around the block once more. It was a cautious start, but it was hugely important for my self-confidence. Going through the small rituals that came with the act of running made it a victory for me and for her. We were both watching closely for any danger signs, even well after we got back home. There were none.

Although we had reached an important first step, I had not yet sorted out where running would fit in my life. That process would take more time.

* * *

Almost as soon as I was discharged, the news from Hamilton about my sister Carolyn took a significant negative turn. She had already been fighting that insidious cancer for more than a year. I don't think any of us were too surprised when it reasserted itself in the summer of 2017. She had already been warned that this was likely to happen. So, just as I turned my attention to getting my life back together, she found herself once more in the fight for her own.

* * *

Running had a way of helping me find answers to questions that I did not even know how to ask. Now that had been snatched away. I felt once more like the teenager, searching for something to belong to. Or maybe something to cling to. I had found running then, or more correctly, running had found me. It had grown into a defining part of my life over many years. Now what was I to do?

By a fortuitous turn, I read a quote from one Thomas Browne, an eighteenth-century Scottish academic. Browne said, "Life is a pure flame, and we live by an invisible sun, burning within us."

Browne's quote stopped me cold. Many things made sense at that moment. A flame was lit in me on that fall day when I followed my teacher's advice and showed up for cross-country practise. I was never a great runner, but by force of will, and by relying on my own personality traits I had stoked the fire and forged myself into a fine and capable athlete. I had achieved success in life, in large part because of the enlightenment that came from engaging my body, mind and spirit through running.

I *had* lived by the heat and light of the invisible sun that burned within me. And what was more, I knew for certain that I could do it again. I could do it for Carolyn, who had inexplicably been struck down with a terrible disease and was fighting gamely against it. I thought about Kathleen, and my mother, who had faced adversity with grace and resilience. I could do the same for them. And for Deb and our sons. But I had to do it for myself first.

After a lot of self-doubt, I came to realize that I already possessed the tools to deal with this setback. Dwelling on what I could not do, what I had lost, would only drag me down further. If I trusted my intuition and kept an open mind—if I let the invisible sun within me shine—then I could figure this out. With the benefit of maturity, I could find some new diversions, or revisit old ones. And if I were diligent in applying myself, I would have reason to expect success. Maybe most importantly, if I stayed humble, I could look past the inevitable missteps that I would make as I tried. If I re-imagined myself as that teenager searching for his niche, who knew what I might find?

* * *

I started close to home and with equipment that I already had close at hand. Since Deb and I were already spending time together walking as part of my rehabilitation, why not take my old Canon film camera that was sitting in a dusty case and shoot some pictures? With the right attitude, this was an opportunity, not a hardship. I began to see things at walking pace that I had missed for so many years while blindly running past.

I learned at once what a satisfying experience it could be to look through a viewfinder in search of something more than snapshots. This was not like using a phone for taking pictures. With the camera—an actual camera—there seemed to be an obligation to slow down and see things more artistically. More elementally. I began looking for form, composition, colour, and pattern. I was no longer seeing things with the same eyes as my 25-year-old self, who at the time was merely imitating one of his heroes, Ansel Adams. Because I had seen more, experienced more—including this physical setback—I started to feel a growing confidence about expressing my own vision. Or maybe I should admit that I was beginning the exploration for my own vision. Even though there was rust to clear away, I had accumulated enough worldly experience to help me shape that vision.

The more pictures I took, the more I wanted to shoot. I eagerly loaded film into my now-vintage cameras. Yes, that was still possible. Here was a self-imposed handicap and an anachronism in our modern digital world, where pictures appeared instantly with the pushing of a button. I remembered the anxious wait for my film to be processed, the ritual of selecting the most promising frames, then the rush that came from editing and cropping them for printing. I found myself wanting to discuss photography with anyone who would listen. With the right attitude, couldn't this be as rewarding as preparing for a goal race? I asked myself how I could have forgotten how much fun this was.

* * *

It happened that running, which had already helped define me once, might play a role in defining the next stage of my life too. In several welcome twists of my story, I confirmed that it could indeed be part of my future. That is why I've started to refer to this period as "my second running life."

In late November 2017, some of my teammates were signed up to race in Calgary's Last Chance Half Marathon. Knowing this, and realizing that the runners would be crossing an attractive new footbridge over the Bow River in the East Village, I suggested to Deb that we take our daily walk in that part of town. Several months after my discharge, we had seen every street in our neighbourhood and we were walking at something approaching our historical pace. My episodes of light-headedness were getting fewer and less severe. I could snap some pictures as the racers crossed the bridge. It would be a nice change of scenery. She agreed.

It was a crisp fall day, a superb day for racing. I got some good photos of the runners as they crossed the arched central span of the bridge before heading further east along the pathway. But the sight of my teammates in race mode, and the realization that I too might have been there if not for the events of that summer, left me feeling dejected. As we walked back to the car, I tried explaining my feelings to Deb. She was as understanding as ever.

I ventured a thought. "Maybe I could look into coaching as a way to stay connected to running."

"You would be a great coach, since you've seen so much," she replied. "Why don't you look into it?"

I did not have to wait long to put the idea into action. The next day, I got a call from Janice. She had heard from the racers that I had been part photographer, part cheerleader the day before.

"How would you like to help out with coaching duties?" she asked. "I think the team would benefit from having you there, given your experience."

Was this a coincidence? Maybe Janice had read my mind. Or maybe Deb had contacted her, to tell her I had expressed an interest in coaching. Whatever the reason, there could only be one possible answer.

"Of course, I'll help out!"

So began a new adventure. I started supervising our interval training sessions on Thursday evenings. With my clipboard in hand, I assumed the role of explainer, encourager, and scribe—otherwise known as assistant coach. In Prince's Island Park for the fall session, we held onto the last bit of daylight and decent weather as long as possible. It had never been easy to give up our wonderful tree-lined circuit for the congested two-lane track around the speedskating rink at the Olympic Oval, which would soon become our winter training base.

At first, I was unsure what value I could add as a coach. I had no formal training that would qualify me for the position. I confided my reluctance to Janice. She asked me to think about the reasons I had entertained the idea of coaching to begin with. There was no question that I had a wealth of knowledge of the sport—the basics of training, the history, the practicalities. I had put in the miles, literally and figuratively. Not only that, but I also had several university degrees, two kids, and ample life experience. In other words, I should be able to trust in a pragmatic approach to coaching. I was over-thinking things.

I welcomed Janice's vote of confidence, but from my own perspective as an athlete I knew that there was much more to being a successful coach. Janice must have recognized that I had some of these attributes. She reminded me why she liked to put new athletes under my wing in workouts. She had trusted me as a safe pair of hands for novice runners. I had always prided myself on executing our workouts well, which for me meant understanding the objective for the session, knowing my paces, and sticking to them. Being disciplined in the execution of a workout was never an issue for me. I had been doing this since tenth grade, after all.

Moreover, I sought to motivate less experienced runners by my example. Since I had started running competitively before some of my teammates were born, I may have been a father figure to them. It made no difference. My teammates had often looked to me to lead them as pacemaker in our interval sessions, and we sometimes joked that I had a good feel for pace because I had started running before watches were invented. For my part, I encouraged a sharing of the workload in training sessions because I knew we all would benefit from having a similar feel. Still, it would be a different experience to be on the sidelines, trying to convey these ideas.

What else did I bring to the coaching role? I'm curious about developments in the sport, but I try not to be swayed too much by faddish training programs, diets, or technology. I think that as athletes we should give ourselves more credit for the investment in time and miles that we have already made. I was well-versed in the amateur athlete's juggling act, the intricate puzzle of balancing work, family life and training schedules. I had been there many times.

Diving in, I began by explaining the workouts, keeping track of interval times, answering questions, and offering what I saw as common-sense advice on training or injury management. And of course, cheerleading. I loved being part of a team, so the easiest part of my coaching role was to be supportive of my teammates. I just had to imagine myself as a teenager, eager to find a place where I belonged. Years later, pulling on a team singlet still felt special to me. Sometimes it only took a few positive words when the going got tough or if the workout seemed too daunting. I recognized when it was time to communicate positive messages, and when it was time to just listen. And that was the most important attribute I brought to this role: a commitment to make a difference for our athletes. If I could not be out on the road with them, I would be with them in spirit as they prepared for race day.

After our long winter session at the Oval, the runners were as anxious as schoolkids for the start of the spring session on Prince's Island. Janice and I discussed individual runner's goals, workout plans and training schedules. She inquired about my own goals. At that point, I still wasn't sure. I was enjoying the coaching gig, but even as I stood in the cold and the wet, with my clipboard getting soaked by heavy spring snow, I began to wonder if I was making any difference in the fortunes of our club runners.

I was gratified when some impressive early results started coming in. This should not have been a surprise, in light of our club's history. After all, these were incredibly competitive athletes, who usually expected to place well in local races, or even on the big stage. In May 2018, a couple of our runners turned in strong performances in the Vancouver Sun Run. I received an email from one of our racers the next day. Vic was a strong runner, whose precocious talent contrasted with his calm, gentle manner and his humility. Maybe I recognized that trait as a common thread between us. I imagined that we would have been well-matched as training partners, were I still in my thirties. While I would have stopped short of saying I had much to do with his results in Vancouver, his note told me a different story.

"You have been there to support us, every workout—urging and motivating us on the sideline when those intervals seemed unbearable!" he said.

Vic's words brought tears to my eyes. And they confirmed that my time and effort had been appreciated. What else could I ask for?

Things built from there. I began to feel accountable for how my teammates did in their target races—from the Boston Marathon to other marathons and to smaller local races. I learned that there was a multiplier effect for a coach. If our athletes met or exceeded their goals, it paid me a dividend I never had earned as a runner. And if they fell short, it caused me to ask what I could have done differently to improve the outcome. The ultimate responsibility on race day was theirs, but I if I could help them see how to respond to certain unforeseen situations, or to feel more confident in their race preparation, then I could serve an important role in their success.

* * *

One other powerful aspect of this experience was the unique position I was in to remind others about the importance of not ignoring any unusual physical symptoms that they observed in themselves or their loved ones. I had been given an opportunity, based on my own experience, to help others.

I thought back to my most satisfying days as a consultant, when I had been able to teach clients something, even something as dry as the inner workings of a refinery or the international trade of oil. Now, my opportunity was to teach people about something that might save their life or the life of a family member. Before all this had started, I would have said I was aware of the symptoms of a stroke. I believed that I could recognize if someone around me were having a stroke. Now, I knew that the range of symptoms could be very wide indeed. The classic signs—loss of control of one side of the body, slurred speech, drooping on one side of the face—relate to strokes in the carotid artery system, which are the most common type. But as I found out, there could be a whole other set of symptoms if a stroke originated in the vertebral arteries.

I learned the power of my message soon after I emailed my friends in Adrenaline Rush to tell them what had happened to me. I reminded them that if they were in any doubt, they should not delay in having symptoms checked out, preferably by calling 911, as I eventually, and reluctantly, had done. Later, after sending out my note, I began to visit with my relieved teammates. Several of them told me that they had taken my advice seriously enough to advise a family member, who had been experiencing unusual health issues, to seek medical care.

If I could be the catalyst for someone getting the help they needed, how could I say no to that?

* * *

Carolyn's disease continued its relentless progress through late 2017 and early 2018, sapping ever more of her energy. I committed to trying to see her more often, which was a challenge, given the constraints on my travelling by air. I knew that nothing could make up for years of our being apart while Deb and I and our sons lived out west. Given what I had just gone through with my hospitalization, I felt I was doing less than I should. We were helpless, being in Calgary and hearing about the ordeal Carolyn was going through with surgery and chemotherapy.

As soon as I had my doctor's approval to travel and felt confident enough to make the trip, I flew to Hamilton to see Carolyn and our mother. They lived only a few blocks apart from each other. I was relieved to see them both. I wasn't sure what I expected to see when I met Carolyn, and she probably felt the same when she saw me. She was in the middle of treatments that left her weak and in a lot of discomfort. She was reduced almost to a shadow, having lost a lot of weight. Her voice was little more than a whisper. I reminded myself that she had always had a quiet demeanour. Maybe there is still hope, I thought. As I expected, Mom was going through hell, right beside Carolyn.

I had long since drifted away from the church, but to the extent that I did any praying during this time, it was for Carolyn, her kids, and my mother. Into this difficult situation stepped my sister Kathleen, my brother Paul and his wife Shelley. Shelley had already been waging her own brave battle with cancer for years. Still, they became like a group of angels for our sick sister. We thanked God for them all.

* * *

A second path to rediscovery opened up for me in early 2018, when Deb announced her interest in running a 5k race. How convenient it was that she would need a training partner, because I was available for the job. It had been several years since her last race and, well, you already know my story. Through the fall and winter, we had done frequent runs of two to three kilometres together. By the time the long winter ended, we had pushed our runs up to as much as five kilometres, so a race at that distance was well within reach. She chose a popular local race, the Stampede 5k, as her goal race. I couldn't help but notice that race day—July 8 — would mark almost exactly one year since my hospitalization.

As race day approached, everything was new again. I went through all the little steps that had previously been second nature. Deb asked me for advice on various topics and together we set out a race plan. I had to keep in mind that this was not about racing, as I had defined it before. Finish times and places were irrelevant. This was about helping Deb reach her goal, and about my regaining another small piece of my former life. I expected that I might get a bit emotional about this last part. I secretly hoped that crossing a finish line would not cause me to burst into tears. That might be embarrassing.

On race day, I had the usual butterflies in my stomach, but this time for a different reason. Our preparation done, we headed to the starting line in the Glenmore Athletic Park, each with something to prove. We hesitated. Where did we belong? My mind flashed back to my last competitive 10k race in May 2017. Then, I had been the picture of a confident athlete as I situated myself at the front of the pack. Now, we were here with another purpose. I thought I had accepted the changes of the past fourteen months. Instead, I felt a helplessness that was new and disorienting. This process was apparently not finished.

In the end, we seeded ourselves on the basis of our estimate of finishing time, opting to slip into an anonymous spot near the middle of the pack. I said a quiet thank you, I'm not sure to whom, that running had become more inclusive, more mainstream, more accepting. While no one other than Deb knew, or even cared, about my reasons for being there, I suddenly felt the weight of what was at stake. I was about to find out if I still had a place at all.

The field was not large, so as soon as the gun went off we were able to find some running room and get settled into our target pace. I offered encouragement and some course guidance. There were many kids in the race, and I did my best to watch out for them too. The first kilometre was a bit slower than we planned, but we were warmed up and running well. We had scouted the route, so we knew it had several small inclines and declines. We adjusted our pace for those. By the third kilometre, our pace had increased. We grabbed some water on the run, which is never easy to do. Deb learned that this was one thing she should have practiced.

As we passed the 4k mark, heading north on Nineteenth Street, I glanced to my right to see runners turning onto the finish straight on the Glenmore Track. I choked up as I realized how much I had missed this experience. I promised myself that there would be more racing in my future. We picked up our pace as we turned onto Fiftieth Avenue. Then we crossed a grassy verge and stepped onto the track. The spongy feel of the synthetic rubber under my feet was instantly familiar. Now we reached the top of the finishing straight. We let ourselves be drawn in by the crowd noise and the announcer's voice. I peeked over and saw that Deb was watching the big clock over the finish line. She was straining to get there before it reached thirty-one minutes. We finished just over, in 31:06. It was a time we could both be satisfied with. We did a recovery walk around the park. As we waited for the results, it sunk in how important this day had been for me—for both of us.

I let myself bask in the energy that was all around us. More than once I had to fight back tears of joy. When the results were posted, we got another boost. Deb had won her age group. She had reached her goal and she was thrilled. I was happy just to be there with her. We met a couple of our Adrenaline Rush teammates at the award ceremony. Scott had won his age group in the 10k, and Annie had run as a pacer in the half marathon. I felt blessed to see them and share our experience with them on this momentous day.

Building on that first small victory, Deb and I continued to test our limits. Janice obliged us with a training program geared to 5k races. Deb took up her side of the bargain by committing to the scheduled workouts. She and I are similarly tenacious and task-oriented, so facing the black and white details of a progressive weekly training program has the effect of focusing our minds on the job at hand. For Deb, it had rekindled a dormant competitive streak. Now it was she who was dragging me along, which was convenient because she could keep an eye on me at the same time.

We have made joint training runs a regular activity, and I am entrusted with the job of timer-in-chief for our weekly interval sessions. There have been more races, most run together, but some as individuals. We have had a measure of our progress, as we have watched our pairs 5k race times drop into the 27- to 28-minute range. My confidence has grown, as we have found a competitive outlet that fits our capabilities. It is ironic that running, which had taken me away from Deb for countless hours during our life together, is now something we can share.

* * *

One day, out of the blue, Carolyn texted me. She had been looking through her old diaries. I suppose she was thinking about her own mortality. She sent me a couple of passages that recounted small, funny details of our family life. Although she could not have known it, she had contacted me on a day when I definitely needed a boost. On one ordinary day in March 1979 "we had roast pork and roast potatoes and creampuffs for dessert, and they were excellent and no complaints," and then she and Kathleen and I had played Monopoly. Another entry described a project I had just finished at university. She had noted how proud she was of her big brother. Carolyn was proud of me! I cried and I laughed as I read those words that she had written so many years earlier, which brought the events they described back to life again through a text.

I saw her once in the spring of 2018. Coincidentally, both of us were in downtown Toronto that day. I had been cleared to fly and was attending a regulatory conference. She was there for a chemotherapy session at the Princess Margaret Hospital. By then, she was pursuing trial treatment options, which were frankly quite limited, and which offered only the slightest hope for a cure. Kathleen had put her own life on hold so she could help get Carolyn from Hamilton to Toronto for the treatments. My first reaction was that Carolyn looked better than she had in our previous visit. And yet, that day (in fact, anytime I talked to her), she was more interested in how I was doing than in talking about herself. Her characteristic empathy reminded me what a peaceful, beautiful soul she was.

It became clear that Carolyn was not going to win her battle with cancer and in September, I got the call we had been dreading. If I wanted to see her one last time, I should make my way to Hamilton as soon as possible. I got there in time to spend a few days with her at the Bob Kemp hospice. It was a blessing to have that last bit of time with her because she was lucid and attentive and talkative the whole time I was there. At times, there were a dozen people in her room. Carolyn drifted in and out of consciousness, but when we suggested it was time to leave, she was adamant.

"I don't want to miss anything," she said simply.

So, we stayed and talked and laughed some more. We even got scolded by the staff for making a bit too much noise. She entertained us with stories of her youth that I had somehow missed. How she and her friend had reluctantly gone horseback riding for a school trip, only to wind up on the two nastiest and most uncooperative horses. How she had tried rock climbing, of all things, with a boy she was briefly interested in. How she had decided it would be a good idea to take the oven door off one day to clean it, only to realize it was not so easy to put back together. Now, her stories were making us all laugh and cry. I was upset with myself for waiting so long to hear them, yet glad that I got to hear them in their last telling.

I returned to Calgary with a heavy heart, knowing that this was likely the last time I would see Carolyn. She died peacefully a couple of days later, on September 12, surrounded by our mother, her children, and the rest of the family in Ontario. It was two weeks after her fifty-third birthday. I shared my thoughts about the precious last three days I had spent with my sister when I spoke at her memorial service later in the month.

Who says life is fair? Even when we know what the end game is for all of us, and that we are all on the same path, it just feels wrong when someone like Carolyn is taken so soon.

* * *

My first instinct as I tried to cope with losing Carolyn was to do what I had always done in painful situations—go for a long solo run and think about her beautiful soul, as I ran alongside the Elbow River or looked out over the Glenmore Reservoir. Now I didn't even have that option. Instead, I felt lost, actually doubly lost. I had lost my sister and I had lost myself. I was still adrift and alone in the ocean.

Then, a couple of months after Carolyn's passing, my mother-in-law Lisa's partner, Andy, died suddenly of a heart attack. Lisa was devastated. They had been together for more than twenty-five years. Andy was the grandfather my kids knew when they were growing up. Deb was once again left to do what she could to help her mother from afar. It was yet another blow. The world was showing itself to be a hard and cruel place.

* * *

Not so many years earlier, starting a running streak had let me find a path forward at a time when I lacked motivation. On a whim, Deb and I signed up for the same holiday challenge at the same running store—the Strides December 2018 Running Streak—soon after Carolyn and Andy had passed away. Coincidentally, it was through this spontaneous act that I found another, and perhaps the most important, path of discovery in my second running life. I had been struggling to come to grips with our recent losses, besides which I was still unsure about my own capabilities. I knew, instinctively, that running would be good therapy.

The parameters were the same as before: run a minimum of one mile a day for the month of December. Several days into the streak, Deb and I were getting ready to head out for a run on a chilly morning. Impulsively, I reached for an old point-and-shoot camera instead of my Garmin watch. I knew she would record the run, so I could get the details from her later. I had been treasuring our recent photo walks, and my idea was to add a photographic element to my running streak. The rules for this impromptu project within a project were simple—I must photograph something interesting that I passed on my run.

While the results from my first run-and-shoot outing would not qualify as fine art, it seemed like a good idea and it stuck. I continued carrying the camera on my runs because it was easy to do and having the camera encouraged me to keep my eyes and my mind open. I started to notice how many worthwhile images I would have missed if I hadn't had the camera—often humorous, sometimes mundane and occasionally beautiful. The process of editing my images later was therapeutic. It helped me capture the essence of what it was like being outside, running, on that day and in that place. I had begun assembling small visual reminders of my return to normalcy.

I came to realize that photography was a proxy for what I was really craving, and that was running without constraints or targets. Without training schedules or goal races. For the first time since being hospitalized, I started feeling confident enough to venture out on my own. And for the first time in decades, since the days that I roamed through King's Forest or Cootes Paradise, I just ran. I ran until I was ready to stop. I walked if I felt like it. I stopped if I saw something worth photographing. The main thing was that I ran without expectations.

I had a much-needed reminder of why running was so special to me. It still was the best expression of human potential. And capturing a little piece of my own potential—again, but for the first time—was a gift that I fully appreciated after the setback I had experienced. I accepted that there were no guarantees about where any of this might lead. There was only the here and now. Personal bests and intermediate split times were irrelevant to me. These were things that rightfully belonged in my past.

At certain rare moments when I was out running and exploring, I felt Carolyn's free spirit beside me. It may have been in the intricate patterns of water and ice on the frozen Bow River, in the hypnotic, tumbling pattern as thousands of starlings appeared in a swarm above my head, in the majestic glow of the rising sun on the Centre Street Bridge. I had been passing scenes like these for years but not seeing them. Now, I knew I had been given another chance and must not miss them. It was almost as if my sister, who had an admirable independent streak, had something to do with this idea. She'd had a way of living in the moment, the way our grandmother had. For so long, I had lived in a different world, a world of self-imposed goals and unforgiving deadlines imposed on me by others. Was Carolyn pointing out these scenes for me, as a way of reminding me that I should start seeing things differently? I could not be sure. At the very least, I knew that my new attitude towards running, and life, was one she would have understood and wholeheartedly approved of.

Equilibrium

I WRITE THESE WORDS FEELING that I have reached a plateau in my recovery. To the outside world, I am back to normal. My medical news has long since moved off any front page.

My mental faculties are intact. As we have done for years, Deb and I can still trade off a Saturday cryptic crossword and she still expects me to hold up my side of things by filling in an answer or two before handing it back to her. Physically, I look the same as I did before, with the exception of one slightly droopy eyelid. For a while, I was interested to see how people who knew me would prepare themselves when they met me for the first time after my hospitalization. Knowing that I'd had strokes, some may have expected to find me physically impaired in some way. I could feel their relief when they would find me looking as they remembered.

I have gotten good at explaining, in my own words, the vascular system and the different types of strokes. I can explain where my arterial occlusion is, usually with a lot of pointing to my head and neck. And I can offer a chemical engineer's explanation of the connection between the subclavian and vertebral arteries. Being able to offer a layman's version has proven helpful when I need to stress to my friends the importance of not ignoring symptoms.

But there have been physical changes, even if they are less obvious than paralysis or loss of motor function. Some days are worse than others. Sometimes I wake up with a strange numbness in my mouth, and with my tongue feeling oddly heavy. Other days I am so confused that I feel like I have woken from a coma. I don't know if these sensations are related to decreased circulation in the back of my head. I have decided to ignore them because they tend to pass quickly.

The most significant physical reminder of my TIA episodes is a minor loss of coordination and balance. After a year or so, I reached what I believe is my new equilibrium. It is a lot closer to my previous functionality than it is to the low point in the hospital. Then, I couldn't even walk around the building without severe vertigo. Now, if I get up during the night, or even when I get up for the day, my legs sometimes don't seem to move the way I want them to. There is a nagging slowness in my legs, as if the signal from my brain to my legs is being delayed ever so slightly. Things still work, just not instantly. The problem usually does not last long once I get myself going. It reminds me of how I felt that morning when we called EMS.

As I go through my day, I get other subtle reminders. They usually come as brief moments of vertigo. If I'm walking down the street and make a sudden turn to look at traffic, a wave of vertigo may hit me. It usually only lasts a few seconds, and it is more disconcerting than anything else. Sometimes it shows up as a feeling that I'm weaving a little as I walk. When this happens, I direct my eyes to a seam on the sidewalk and force myself to stay parallel to it, or I walk close to a wall using a hand to steady myself. These are not surprising outcomes, when I consider the residual damage in the part of my brain that controls these functions.

Even now, I go through checklists of my physical functions.

Am I able to walk in a straight line or am I veering off to the right? Are my eyes working as they should? Is my head clear or has the vertigo returned? Did I see something unusual in my field of vision? Was that feeling in my neck an ordinary muscle spasm or was it something more serious?

When I explain these things to Deb, she tends to downplay them a little. She is right that I'm not as young as I used to be, so it may not be a surprise that I would occasionally have trouble getting going in the morning. If I'm honest with myself, I often felt that way the day after a long run or interval session. Still, she can't be inside my body, and despite the concessions to advancing years, I know what I know. There have been some permanent physical changes, even if they are minor.

* * *

My sleep habits have changed too. I don't know whether that is due to the lingering effects of the blocked artery or due to side effects of my daily drug cocktail. Gone are the nights where I could push my mind and body well past midnight if a project called for me to do that. Now I find myself nodding off by 10 P.M., getting almost overwhelmed by feelings of fatigue if I try to fight it. There are no more late-night television talk shows for me.

The fatigue that weighs on me in the evening means that I am usually asleep as soon as I hit the pillow, and that the early hours of the night bring deep sleep, maybe deeper than I've ever experienced before. If I'm truthful, it's deeper than what I'm comfortable with. Now, when I wake up, as I usually do after a few hours, it is often with that same confused feeling of waking up as if from a coma.

I often wake abruptly in the early hours of the morning, and then endure long stretches before I can get back to sleep. Because I have come to expect this pattern, I let myself lie awake by anticipating it and not getting frustrated. If I'm lucky, I make use of the time, by settling into positive thoughts. For a while this was helpful in getting myself organized to write this book. Often, I find myself in some kind of contact with Carolyn or Dad or others who have gone before me. I don't know if I'd call this prayer, but it is a connection with them, and that makes it pleasant and satisfying.

Sometimes, I just lie there, not thinking much about anything. This is the middle ground, and I can live with it too. When Deb was working and trying to get a decent sleep before her early morning start, I would stay as still as possible so as not to bother her, but I suspected she was often lying there awake beside me. I would wonder what things she was thinking about. Maybe they were the same things I grappled with as I lay awake.

Since my hospitalization, I avoid lying on my left side, because then I can distinctly feel the blood flow pumping through the vertebral artery—my one good one—at the back of my neck. With each pulse, I can feel the blood being sent into my brain. It doesn't hurt, but it is too much of a reminder. I think I always felt that pulse, but now it has taken on a more ominous meaning. If I'm in a positive frame of mind, I marvel at this process repeating itself forty or fifty times a minute, and I feel quite lucky. On the nights when I'm in a darker place, it's a different story. On those nights, I don't feel lucky at all. In the stages of grief model, this one—depression—is the place I'd rather not get stalled. These are the nights where the precariousness of my position starts to get the better of me.

I think about those tiny collateral arteries doing the job of the blocked vertebral, and I wonder how long it will be before they expire. Dr. Demchuk had mused about the worst-case scenario, a massive basilar stroke brought on by the lack of blood flow through my single, compromised vertebral artery. It doesn't take a lot of medical expertise to imagine what that might look like. All I need to do is think about the functions controlled by this part of my brain and imagine them stopping cold. I have the list memorized by now—difficulty with balance and coordination, vertigo, double vision or loss of vision, problems with swallowing and talking, numbness, weakness, memory loss, incontinence. The list goes on. Balance and vision symptoms alerted me to the fact that something was wrong in the first place. I think back to that unexplained, out-of-body fainting episode in my office. Then the TIAs that followed, each one seemingly more bizarre than the last, were a prelude to more serious outcomes.

As I lie there, I think back to that night in the hospital, when I clung to the words of the late-night television left on by another patient, just before I sank into another round of TIAs. Then, the television was not an annoyance, but a lifeline. Now, I concentrate on the sounds in my bedroom—the furnace, my bedside humidifier—listening for any minute change and wondering whether it is an artefact caused by a momentary dip in the blood flow to my brain, or whether it is real. I listen for Deb's breathing, reassuring me like a safe harbour of familiar sound.

Yes, I'm still here, I say to myself. I'm fine, for now.

The thought of that strange black curtain being pulled in front of my eyes again—this time permanently—sends a shiver through me, and I suddenly feel very alone, even with Deb beside me. In the dark, I open each eye in turn to make sure that it can still make out the familiar shapes in my room—the window, the doorframe, the lamp. Yes, they are still there, and I can see them.

* * *

I sometimes find myself spinning what-if cases, like well-worn pathways in my mind. I imagine how differently things might have turned out if I had suffered a catastrophic stroke in the middle of Stage 8 during the K-100 Relay in June 2017. How long would it have taken for anyone to get to me as I lay on the side of the road? How long until I was delivered to the hospital in Calgary? And what would have been left of my brain by the time they figured out what had happened to me?

Or what if I had been struck down while doing that exhausting interval workout in Central Park in New York City on my own, without any identification and without a phone? Where would I have ended up, and in what condition?

I think about what might have happened had I not woken up when Deb got up in the middle of the fateful night that led to my hospital stay. She would have gone to work just like she did every other workday. I believe something forced me to wake up that night and tell her about my TIA. What if that had never happened?

I know it does me absolutely no good to spin these thoughts. It's just that I can't control where my mind takes itself. I think this process originates in the same place as the stream of consciousness that used to occupy me on long runs. Then, my mind would go where it wanted to go. I thrived on that feeling, that I could use my running time as an opportunity to be alone with my thoughts. I could solve problems or come up with new ways of looking at issues. That's why I preferred to run without music or gadgets. I wanted my mind to run as my body ran. Now, it seems I have trouble turning that switch off.

There is another scenario that has confounded me since my diagnosis and at the same time given me hope for the future. What if I hadn't been pushing my system for years to build me a system of collateral arteries? I believe that the pain I felt in my left shoulder and neck between 2010 and 2012 while training was caused by my vascular system building bypasses around a growing arterial blockage. At the time, I saw physiotherapists and even a chiropractor. If those bypasses had not been built, my fate likely would have been sealed once the flow in my artery became completely blocked.

Since lying in my hospital bed, and for almost a year afterwards, I experienced pain in the same spot. Even now, if I push myself too hard on a run, or if I try to do too much around the house, I feel the overexertion first as a nagging soreness in that spot. No one will be able to confirm it, but I'm convinced that this pain is due to the collaterals growing in size as they adapt to their expanded—actually, vital—role. My doctors predicted that this would happen. Dr. Demchuk even speculated that the dead leg in my vertebral artery would close off on its own, reducing the risk of any further embolic strokes. If these things are true, they confirm what a miraculous machine the human body is.

I could drive myself crazy thinking about all of this. All I know for sure is that I am fortunate because I still have all my motor functions, all my senses, and all my mental faculties. I have lost some brain matter though. That was clear from looking at the array of white spots—dead spots—on an MRI scan of my brain. At this point, Deb may joke that I didn't have any spare brain to lose, but we both know that it could have been much, much worse.

* * *

And how should I face the future? With my foundation shaken by the events of the last five years, that is not an easy question to answer. In the immediate aftermath, I felt like an earthquake survivor, picking through the rubble of what was my house. I had to keep reminding myself that I was alive, but with the knowledge that nothing could ever be the same again. I was in shock, unable to even think straight.

I have accepted that I will never make sense of what happened to me. I believe it happened for a reason, even if I may never know what that reason is. Slowly, surely, though, I have come to terms with my situation. I can begin to imagine a real future. What is important, as the old saying goes, is that I live each day as though it is my last.

Restoring everything to normal, as least as I would like to define it, seems unlikely, without some medical solution that I am not aware of right now. Perhaps the doctors will surprise me, and I will one day be able to do a demanding workout with my teammates, in the late stages of preparation for a goal race. Probably not, though. The more likely scenarios are considerably more sedate, but far from terrible. I see myself doing many of the things that I once took for granted. I can run, albeit at a slower pace. I've confirmed with Dr. Demchuk that I can play golf, although my discussion with him reminded me of the joke about the patient asking his doctor if he will be able to play the piano after his operation.

"Sure," the doctor says. And the guy responds by saying, "Great. I couldn't do it before." That seems to describe my golf game perfectly.

Rather than dwell on what I cannot do, I can be encouraged by the progress I've made since my hospital stay. Whereas then, I could not make it around the building without feeling a wave of vertigo, I can celebrate that it is now rare for me to feel that way, even for a few seconds. I have not had any more attacks, and I have long since stopped keeping an informal list of tasks that I can still do. I can do anything I am interested in doing.

Rather than focusing on how tenuous my situation is, I can remind myself that none of us, no one, knows what our future holds. There are innumerable scenarios that we could imagine in our own dark moments. If we are sensible, though, we dedicate ourselves to more productive pursuits. That describes me, most of the time.

Rather than think about those whispery thin collateral arteries doing the job of my blocked left vertebral—the angiogram video playing on a permanent loop of fill, fill, fill, pump—I can choose to think about newly fortified arteries doing their job well, and for many years to come.

Then I remind myself of the tools that equipped me to get to where I am today. Be curious, be diligent, and be humble. These seem, more than ever before, to be my rules to live by. After all, I may find myself pursuing activities that I am not proficient at. I will fail at many things, but I may also succeed at a few. I hope to discover talents that I never knew I had. I feel like I'm back to where I was as that teenager, more than four decades ago, searching for his niche among an infinite range of options—sports, careers, hobbies. If that is the worst that comes out of this adventure, I should be looking forward with optimism and hope.

The best news of all is that I can keep running on my list. I have found a unique way to keep moving forward—I am on a path that lets me help others to pursue their goals in the sport, includes the love of my life in a way that had never been realistic before, and frees me to enjoy the intrinsic benefits of running without obsessing over times and paces.

A Running Life in Perspective

I WALKED TO THE STARTING line of a race on a glorious May morning, as I had done so many times before. The events of that morning would have been indistinguishable from those of just about any other race day. On that morning, I applied the necessary commitment to the task at hand, facilitated by hours of resolute and purposeful training. But I also brought a sense of renewed dedication to the sport I loved.

It was something I thought about often, this connection I had with running. After all, I had been living the life of an amateur athlete for more than four decades. If I had been pressed, though, my attempts to verbalize what that meant would likely have fallen short of the mark. I have enjoyed many benefits from my involvement in the sport. Not least among these is perspective—the ability to see things in their proper context. But I have had time for proper reflection lately, and I see clearly that this attachment—more accurately, my relationship—transcends the boundaries of amateur sport, since it has been an integral part of my existence for so long.

Running had accompanied me through all the notable achievements of my life. More than that, it had enabled me to reach those heights. It had given me the means to realize my full potential, personally and professionally, working with and through facets of my personality. In the same way, it had allowed me to find a path to solace, on those occasions where life's prescribed rituals seemed to be inadequate. It had enriched my relationships and pushed me to test my own limitations. In short, I would not be the person I am today without running.

None of this was in my mind on that sunny spring morning. Things were still simple and uncomplicated. I was looking forward to 2017 as a year of change and of new challenges, limited (or so I thought) to the realm of race distances and training plans—questions neatly defined in terms of kilometres and seconds. I could not possibly have known on that morning the direction and extent of the changes to come. My life was about to be transformed in ways that I could not have imagined. Initially, the transformation would only be hinted at in brief glimpses. It should not have been surprising that those early signs would have been interpreted by a runner to be the result of anything other than what they truly were. They could have been the result of too quick a pace under race conditions, or not drinking enough water on a hot day, or of not taking adequate recovery after a strenuous workout.

Soon enough, when the full magnitude of the problem could no longer be ignored or rationalized away, it would swallow up my relationship with running. It would threaten much more than my involvement with amateur sport, whatever importance I might have attached to that. It would threaten life as I knew it and leave my prospects in doubt. From the depths of my denial and anger, laying in the stroke unit, while the TIAs inflicted damaging blows and the doctors searched for a response, it was unclear what kind of life I would be left with. Or whether I would ever leave that place to try and have a life.

Until those dark days, I had never given much thought to my

mortality. Maybe that is the fate of the lapsed Catholic, as a natural reaction to too much emphasis on the next life. Maybe I felt my running resume had conferred on me some type of exemption from such worries. Or maybe it is that this all happened too early, before I was ready to consider any of these scenarios for myself. If I'm totally honest, I had let the years slip by me faster than I would have liked. Besides the impetus imposed by my hospitalization, I have recently passed the age of sixty, so those numbers are getting harder to ignore. There are some milestones that have more effect on the psyche than others. This is one of those.

Slowly, the clouds did dissipate, and a path forward to life became clearer. I seem to have retained my mental abilities, and I eventually regained most of the physical capabilities I had lost. I am finding the confidence to push my boundaries once again. I have stopped worrying about the what-ifs of my past and shifted my emphasis to the why-nots of my future.

And what about that future? As the events of 2017 recede into memory, I have been able to compartmentalize them and all that has happened since, as a reminder. A wake-up call, if you like. To the extent I did think about what my future looked like, it was in the form of an idealized self-portrait. Even if there were not less runway in front of me than behind, I had every reason to expect many more quality years. At eighty-five, I expected to be fit and of sound mind. It would have gone without saying that running was to be a part of my life every day until then. Indeed, running was in some ways the point of it all. Getting older without being able to run would render life unlivable, or so I thought. I would continue running and racing, because competitive running and all that came with it was what grounded me and gave my life purpose. By continuing to train and race, I would know I was alive. Literally, competitive running was life.

Now, I know that that picture is likely to remain a dream. I have no assurances about any part of it. I do not know what my odds are of reaching sixty-five, let alone eighty-five. If I do make it to an age marked by one or other arbitrary number, I do not know that I will arrive there fit, strong, and mentally sharp. Thanks to an inch of faulty plumbing in the back of my neck, just above the level of my collarbone, a day may come that I am unable to race, or even walk. I may not be able to make sense of what I see or hear. Those are scary prospects, to be sure.

There are a couple of thoughts that keep me from wallowing in self-pity. One is a simple fact that I have now accepted. None of us, however devoted we might be to fitness regimens or diets or self-help books, gets a guarantee about their future or what it will look like. No one has ever had such a guarantee. The end game is the only thing we know for sure. Everything else is conjecture.

And I have relied on another thought to console myself. Even if my current capabilities are reduced, I have the good fortune of being able to make choices that will add value to my life and the lives of those around me. I am blessed to have opportunities for alternative avenues of learning and personal expression. Through photography, or writing, or relearning to play the guitar, or any number of as-yet undefined activities, I can challenge myself and maybe give comfort to others. Even in that most familiar territory of all, running, I have found several ways to expand my involvement, and experience more joy than I otherwise might have expected. There is still a why for choosing to live. I am only beginning to define the how, and it is an exhilarating prospect.

And so, there is another picture, a real one, that has replaced the nostalgic and highly uncertain one of my dreams. It tells a better story, and hints at a more realistic future. It is a picture taken at the finish line of the 2019 Dino Dash, a race that supports young track athletes at the University of Calgary. These are the same athletes I often see at the Olympic Oval, as we each go through our interval training sessions on cold winter evenings. Sharing the track with them never fails to make me feel young again too.

As has become our standard practice, Deb and I ran the 5k race together and watched out for each other. The race happened to fall on the date of our thirty-fifth wedding anniversary. It was slightly more than two years on from my hospitalization. If I do say so myself, we make quite an attractive couple, posing at the finish line in our matching team outfits. We are apparently undeterred by the open jaws of a life-sized inflatable T. Rex, the Dino team mascot, just behind us. Rather, we both look relaxed and happy, although perhaps for different reasons. Deb is happy because she has just finished second in her age group. I am pleased about that, of course, but also because I have won another chance at life, a life that includes running, and its several paths to rediscovery. We are clearly thrilled to be there, together. And maybe the T. Rex is there to remind us of the unknown risks that lurk in our future. But as long as I am still able to run, and have Deb beside me, I feel I will be equal to those challenges.

I know what my task is going forward. I must focus on being the best version of myself, every minute I have left. If one door closes, I need to find another and tear it down. I must let my invisible sun burn at its brightest. By doing so, I can demonstrate to myself, to those that have gone before me, and to those that are still traveling with me on this journey that I am choosing to defy the odds. I will do this despite having the odds inevitably and forever stacked against me. But this is not selfish or foolish. It is the truest expression of caring and love.

And with that, it is time for a run.

Acknowledgements

I am indebted to many people who have contributed, in all sorts of ways, to enriching my life as an amateur athlete. Because I have been about as amateur as it gets, and because the timeframe of my competitive running career is rather long, recognition of my debt of gratitude is necessarily broad and covers contributions that go well beyond the competitive sphere. Suffice to say, I am thankful for the support that has led to success in all aspects of my life, of which running has been the catalyst. One thing is certain—I have been extraordinarily blessed in my journey. This has been a phenomenal adventure so far and it appears likely to remain interesting as I go forward.

Starting where I rightly should, I thank my mother Carm and my late father Ken for giving me the best possible start in life. I could not begin to do proper justice to the value of your example if I started to enumerate the ways you have helped me. Thanks too, to the rest of my family, my dear sister Kathleen, my beloved sister Carolyn (gone far too soon), my brother Paul, my grandparents. You made the start of my story read like a novel, which is a good thing. The story of my early years may even be the genesis of another book some day. To my family by marriage, first my wonderful in-laws, Lisa and Kurt, and then by good fortune, Andy, thank you for treating me as your son. I am also indebted to my late sister-in-law Shelley and my brother-in-law Tom. My cousin Brenda deserves thanks for her many suggestions throughout this project, and for always being willing to talk about books.

Once the flame was lit and my way to the starting line—literal and figurative—was illuminated, I began the apprenticeship that the sport of competitive running seems uniquely able to offer. Along the way I have been fortunate to share the road with many great running partners and teammates. Thanks to all of you for helping the miles pass with humour and a sense of shared commitment. I cannot possibly name everyone, but one person deserves special mention. Mahedi, you are a true friend, and I will always consider it an honour to run beside you. To everyone in Adrenaline Rush, it has been a privilege to run with you, and lately, to help motivate you. I will let you in on a little secret: you motivate me just as much.

I would not have managed to squeeze as much joy and satisfaction from the sport of running as I have, and I'm sure I would not have stuck with it this long, were it not for the help and guidance of wonderful coaches. Thank you, Mr. Menegon and Mr. James (not his real name) for making sure I made it cross-country practice on that fateful day so many years ago. Thanks also to Calgary legends Gord and Ray, Mahedi (again), and of course Janice, for all you have done to keep the flame burning. And for fixing the worst of my running posture, too. You each have a share in my modest PB's. On a related note, to Gord and Jeremy Deere, I value all you do to support the local running community. You are instrumental in keeping our passion alive.

To Dr. Demchuk, Dr. Menon, the amazing doctors and staff at the Stroke Prevention Clinic, and the many unsung heroes of the tenth floor Foothills Stroke Unit—the nurses, the orderlies, the cleaning staff—I would not be here if it weren't for you. I owe you all more than I could ever repay. In the same light, I owe an extra debt of gratitude to Dr. Stephen Wood, who for a few tense days in July 2017 managed to simultaneously be a teammate, an independent medical advisor, and a confidant. You are the best, fast Steve!

To those colleagues who have proven themselves to be so much more, know that you are valued more than I could put into words. For my friends and former partners at Purvin & Gertz, particularly my mentors who showed me what being a consultant was all about, I can only marvel at what we accomplished, together. Those really were the days. Thanks, Phil, for helping me sharpen my vision and find my voice. And to Murray and Shane and Ron, it is definitely my turn to buy next time we find ourselves at Weeds Café.

I am indebted to those who helped me with the process of preparing the book. Thanks to Rona Altrows for her excellent editing assistance. I am fortunate to have talented and generous neighbours —Lori Beattie, Susan and Kelly Wright —who tolerated my many questions as they guided me through the world of book publication. Extra thanks are due to Kelly for the first-class book design. Thanks also to Martin Parnell, Teresa Wong, Meg Braem, Michael Brennan and Murray (again) for your help and support.

And that leaves only three people to thank—the most important ones. Deb, you have been beside me for most of this journey. In the good times and in the bad times, you have been my anchor and my inspiration. Everything positive that I've thought worthy of including in this memoir is your accomplishment as much as mine. Thanks for putting up with my seemingly unavoidable prerace grouchiness all those years. We belong together, and that explains why we have achieved so much together. Our two greatest achievements, Matt and Dan, are both now well on their way due in the largest part to your guiding hand. And guys, as I say thanks for making my life complete, I will offer you the same advice I have tried to follow myself—be ever curious, diligent, and humble. My love to all three of you.

About the Author

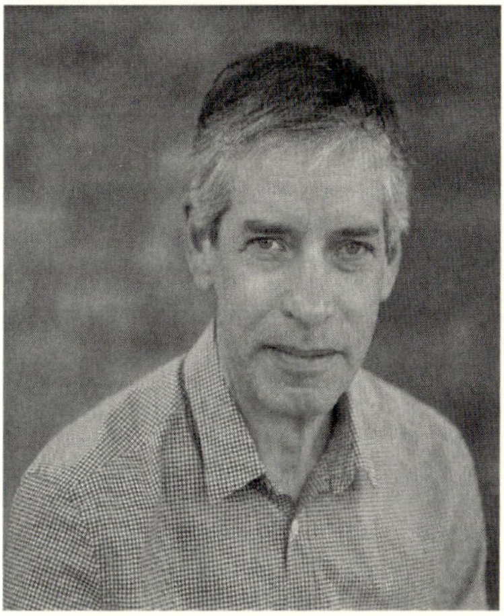

© Photo by Gord MacPherson

Steven Kelly is a semi-retired chemical engineer and a dedicated amateur runner, who has competed in road races for almost fifty years. He grew up in a working-class city in Ontario. Telling the story of his recovery from a series of strokes has allowed Steve to pursue another of his lifelong interests, non-fiction writing. He lives in Calgary, Alberta, and while he still enjoys running along the river pathways, it is now at a slower pace and usually includes photography. Steve and his wife Deborah enjoy travelling and reading. They have two grown sons.